LECTURE NOTES ON
DISEASES OF THE EAR
NOSE AND THROAT

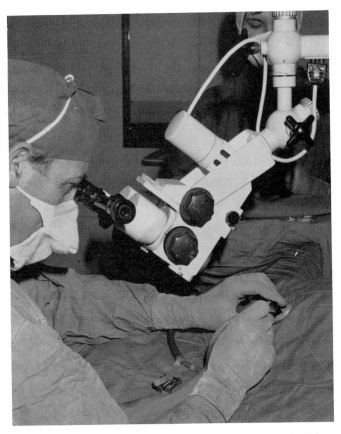

Frontispiece. A binocular operating microscope (in this case one of the Zeiss Otoscopes), is now used for many aural and laryngeal operations.

LECTURE NOTES ON
DISEASES OF THE EAR
NOSE AND THROAT

E. H. Miles Foxen
F.R.C.S., D.L.O.

Consulting Surgeon
Ear, Nose and Throat Department
Westminster Hospital

FIFTH EDITION

BLACKWELL SCIENTIFIC PUBLICATIONS
OXFORD LONDON EDINBURGH
BOSTON MELBOURNE

© 1961, 1968, 1972, 1976, 1980 by
Blackwell Scientific Publications
Editorial offices:
Osney Mead, Oxford, OX2 oEL
8 John Street, London, WC1N 2ES
9 Forrest Road, Edinburgh, EH1 2QH
52 Beacon Street, Boston,
    Massachusetts 02108, USA
214 Berkeley Street, Carlton,
    Victoria 3053, Australia

First published 1961
Reprinted 1962, 1965, 1967
Second edition 1968
Reprinted 1970, 1971
Third edition 1972
Reprinted 1975
Fourth edition 1976
Reprinted 1978
Fifth edition 1980

Printed and bound in Great Britain
at the Alden Press, Oxford.

DISTRIBUTORS

USA
    Blackwell Mosby Book Distributors
    11830 Westline Industrial Drive
    St Louis, Missouri 63141

Canada
    Blackwell Mosby Book Distributors
    120 Melford Drive, Scarborough
    Ontario, M1B 2X4

Australia
    Blackwell Scientific Book
    Distributors
    214 Berkeley Street, Carlton
    Victoria 3053

British Library
Cataloguing in Publication Data

Foxen, Eric Harry Miles
    Lecture notes on diseases of the ear, nose
    and throat.—5th ed.
    1. Otolaryngology
    I. Title
    616.2'1   RF46

ISBN 0-632-00652-8

CONTENTS

PREFACE TO FIFTH EDITION

ALTHOUGH the fourth edition has been thoroughly revised, the object of this book remains the same—to act as a guide to beginners by laying emphasis on important conditions and on the principles of otolaryngological practice.

Even during the last four or five years enormous advances have been made in the field of audiology, and although much of this particular discipline is far beyond the scope of a small introductory book it remains a fact that the House Officer should at least be aware of what tests are available for further investigation in a particular case of deafness. For this reason the advanced methods are mentioned and the interested reader is given guidance regarding further reading in more detailed textbooks.

It might be argued that there was no point in retaining the essay questions set between the years 1958–66. Nevertheless, the author firmly believes that the best way of revising for any examination in essay or multiple choice form is to test oneself with questions which have been set previously.

Westminster Hospital, London SW1   E. H. MILES FOXEN
1980

PREFACE TO FIRST EDITION

THIS book is intended for the undergraduate medical student and the house officer. It is hoped that, though elementary, it will also prove of use to the general practitioner.

Many conditions encompassed within the so-called 'specialist' subjects are commonly seen in general practice, and the practitioner is therefore obliged to be familiar with them. He is not asked to perform complex aural operations, or even to be acquainted with their details, but he is expected to appreciate the significance of headache supervening in otitis media, to treat epistaxis, and to know the indications for tonsillectomy.

Emphasis has therefore been laid on conditions which are important either because they are common or because they call for investigation or early treatment. Conversely, some rare conditions and specialized techniques have received but scant attention, whilst others have been omitted, for the undergraduate should be protected from too much 'small print', which will clutter his mind, and which belongs more properly to post-graduate studies.

The study of past examination questions should be an integral part of the preparation for any examination, and students are strongly advised to 'work-up' the examination questions at the end of the book. Time spent in this occupation will certainly not be wasted, for the questions refer, in every case, to the fundamentals of the specialty.

E. H. MILES FOXEN

ACKNOWLEDGEMENTS

I AM most grateful to Dr Peter Hansell's Department of Medical Illustrations at Westminster Hospital and Medical School for the illustrations in this book. Almost all the line drawings were executed by the late Jill Hassell. The numerous illustrations which she prepared with such ready cooperation remain a tribute to the memory of a devoted Medical Artist.

I am also grateful to Down Bros. and Mayer & Phelps Ltd who have made available certain blocks for illustration of instruments, to Alfred Peters & Sons Ltd for the photograph of their Clinic Audiometer and to Keeler Instruments Ltd for the photograph of two of their Otoscopes.

I am indebted to the authorities of the Universities of Cambridge, London and Oxford, and the Committee of Management of the Examining Board in England for permission to reproduce questions which have been set in final examinations in surgery.

Finally, I must pay tribute with grateful thanks to the care and patience exercised by my secretaries, Mrs Dulcie Fletcher—who prepared the manuscript for the first edition—and Miss Wendy Kaye whose meticulous attention to detail has helped to launch subsequent editions and reprints.

CHAPTER 1

THE EAR: SOME APPLIED ANATOMY

The auricle, composed of cartilage and closely adherent perichondrium and skin, is developed from six tubercles. Fistulae and accessory auricles may develop if these tubercles fail to fuse.

The external auditory meatus, about one inch in length, has a skeleton of cartilage in its outer third (where it contains hairs and ceruminous glands) and bone in its inner two-thirds. The skin of the inner part is exceedingly thin, adherent and *sensitive*. At the medial end of the meatus there is a depression, the antero-inferior recess, in which *wax, debris or foreign bodies may lodge.*

The tympanic membrane (Fig. 1) is composed of three layers, skin, fibrous tissue and mucous membrane, the middle layer being absent in the pars flaccida. The drum-head is set at an angle of 55° with the floor of the meatus, and in the infant this angle is considerably less.

The tympanic cavity, though tall (15 mm) and long antero-posteriorly (15 mm), is extremely *narrow*, the tympanic membrane being only 2 mm from the promontory, a point to bear in mind when performing myringotomy. The upper part of the cavity—the epitympanic recess—contains the head of the malleus and the body of the incus, and communicates posteriorly via the aditus with the mastoid antrum (Fig. 2). The latter

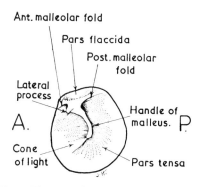

Fig. 1. The normal tympanic membrane (left).

I

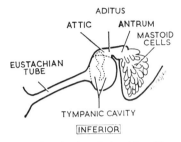

SUPERIOR

ADITUS
ATTIC   ANTRUM
MASTOID
CELLS
EUSTACHIAN
TUBE

TYMPANIC CAVITY

INFERIOR

Fig. 2. The tympanic cavity showing its relationship to Eustachian tube and mastoid cells. The tympanic membrane and malleus are indicated by broken lines.

has an important surface marking on the temporal bone postero-superiorly to the external meatus. This is the **suprameatal triangle of Macewen,** which is bounded above by the posterior root of the zygoma, behind by a vertical line dropped from the zygomatic root to the posterior wall of the meatus, and anteriorly by a line joining the first two and tangential to the postero-superior meatal wall (Fig. 3).

The anatomical features of the medial wall of the tympanic cavity are crowded; lateral semicircular canal, facial nerve, oval and round windows and promontory being within a few millimetres of each other (Fig. 4). An injury of this region, therefore, is likely to have devastating results—facial paralysis, labyrinthitis, deafness, and, perhaps, meningitis.

The Eustachian tube, about one and a half inches in length, is more horizontal and relatively wider in the infant than the adult. Thus in

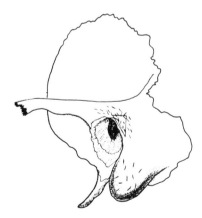

Fig. 3. The suprameatal triangle of Macewen.

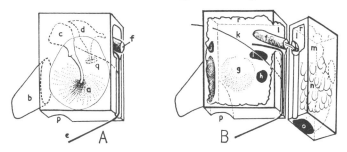

Fig. 4. Diagram of the middle ear cavity and some of its immediate relations. In A the tympanic membrane is present. In B the tympanic membrane and ossicles have been removed and the mastoid antrum and cells swung medially in order to show the relationship of facial nerve, lateral semicircular canal and aditus.

a. Tympanic membrane. *b*. Eustachian tube. *c*. Malleus. *d*. Incus. *e*. Facial nerve. *f*. Lateral semicircular canal. *g*. Promontory. *h*. Round window. *i*. Oval window. *j*. Canal for tensor tympani. *k*. Chorda tympani. *l*. Aditus. *m*. Mastoid antrum. *n*. Mastoid cells. *o*. Lateral sinus. *p*. Internal carotid artery. *q*. Stapes. *r*. Tegmen.

infantile gastro-enteritis *vomitus* can enter the tympanic cavity with ease.

The facial nerve is a subcutaneous and relatively unprotected structure in children of under two. *Post-aural incisions must be kept high* (Fig. 5).

The mastoid cells vary considerably in development. In a temporal bone they may extend into the squama, the zygoma, and along the petrous to its tip. Mastoiditis in such a bone will be extensive.

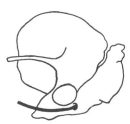

Fig. 5. The unprotected facial nerve in the infant.

CHAPTER 2
CLINICAL EXAMINATION
OF THE EAR

MEDICAL students by tradition are taught to use the head-mirror for the clinical examination of patients attending ear, nose and throat departments. This is desirable, and with a little practice most undergraduate students acquire skill in inspecting the nose and pharynx and even the nasopharynx and larynx. But in order to interpret what he sees in the ear with the head-mirror and simple aural speculum, the average student requires not weeks but months of practice, and for this reason it is better for him to master the use of the **electric otoscope** (auriscope) from the outset, for this is the instrument he will probably use in general practice (Fig. 6).

When students commence clinical work on their general firms and express a desire to examine their patients' ears, they are not infrequently handed an otoscope which conforms to the following standards:

1   The battery is 30–40 per cent efficient.
2   The bulb-carrier has become bent, and the feeble glimmer emanating is not even directed out of the end of the speculum, but rather to one side (Fig. 7).
3   The speculum chosen is either too large or too small (usually the latter). It may also have unnecessarily thick walls.

It is not surprising that the unfortunate novice attributes his failure to see the tympanic membrane to his own shortcomings rather than to the inadequacy of the instrument, and, after a time, comes to regard otologists as being gifted either with abnormally acute vision or an unduly vivid imagination. This is not the case. With a good instrument and a little instruction, the veriest tyro may examine the tympanic membrane with ease, but he must first make sure of the following basic requirements:

1   The battery is well up to standard.
2   The main beam of light is directed out of the end of the speculum.
3   The speculum is the largest which can be inserted without causing pain.

Having obtained a satisfactory instrument, remember the following points:

4

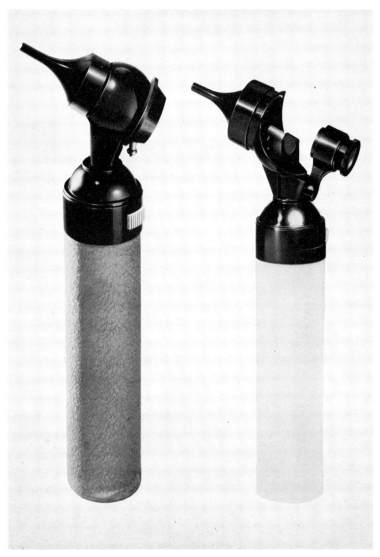

Fig. 6. Electric otoscopes. The two excellent models illustrated are manufactured by Keeler Instruments Ltd.

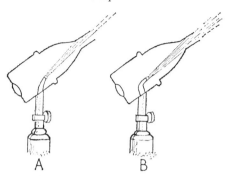

Fig. 7. A common condition of otoscopes; usually the result of trauma. The bulb holder in A has been bent.

1 The external meatus is very sensitive to pressure. Insert the speculum gently and not too far.

2 The meatus is sensitive to temperature change. If, in winter, your instrument case has just been extracted from the boot of your car, the speculum may be very cold. Warm it gently.

3 There is usually a kink in the meatus. Draw the auricle gently upwards and backwards (downwards and backwards in infants), in order to straighten the meatus.

4 If the inserted speculum is held in exactly the same position throughout the examination, only a limited area of the tympanic membrane will be seen. The angle at which the speculum is inserted into the meatus must be varied.

5 Make use of the small rubber bulb, which should be provided with all instruments. With it the mobility of a normal tympanic membrane may be readily demonstrated.

The appearance of the normal external meatus varies within fairly wide limits, particularly as regards diameter, shape, and the growth of hair. Hairs are limited to the outer, membranous part, but may be very numerous. Wax may be present, and, if so, must be removed before the inspection can be completed.

Normal tympanic membranes also vary to some extent both in colour, translucency, size, shape and inclination to the sagittal and horizontal planes. The student is therefore advised to examine as many normals as possible, for such an occupation, though somewhat arduous, is the only means of acquiring the ability to recognize the abnormal without hesitation.

CHAPTER 3
TESTING THE HEARING

CLINICAL testing of the hearing is a process involving three definite stages, which should always be carried out in the same order.

Stage I. Simple assessment of the degree of deafness.

Stage II. Tuning fork tests.

Stage III. Audiometry.

SIMPLE ASSESSMENT OF THE
DEGREE OF DEAFNESS

The patient is asked to sit in a chair, facing the wall, at one end of the room, and to occlude the deafer ear by pressing with his finger against the tragus. He is instructed to repeat after the examiner whatever the latter says.

The examiner, commencing at the far end of the room, whispers test words or numbers, and approaches until the patient is able to repeat the words accurately. If moderate or severe deafness is present, it may be necessary for the examiner to employ 'Conversational Voice'. The distance from patient to examiner is now noted, and might be expressed, for example, in a slightly deaf person as W.V. (whispered voice) at 5′ or in a case of severe deafness, C.V. (conversational voice) at 6″.

Now the deafer ear is tested in the same way, the better ear being occluded.

There is a trap for the unwary. Suppose it is found on this preliminary testing that a gross difference in the hearing acuity of the two ears is present, e.g. R. Ear W.V. 12′: L. Ear C.V. 2′, it is quite possible that the more deaf ear is, in fact, very much more deaf than at first presumed. It may, in fact, be totally deaf. The reason is that though the patient appeared to hear C.V. at 2′ with the L. Ear, he was, in fact, hearing the voice with his R. Ear, simple occlusion of the meatus being an inadequate method of suppressing hearing in a good ear.

A simple method of avoiding this error is by introducing the measure of masking the better ear by applying to it a Bárány noise apparatus whilst the deafer ear is tested by C.V. The noise emitted by the clockwork

7

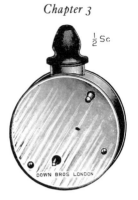

Fig. 8. Bárány noise apparatus.

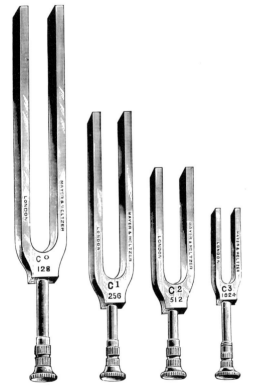

Fig. 9. Tuning forks. The 512 c.p.s. fork is the most useful.

mechanism of this little machine effectively occupies the attention of the better cochlea (Fig. 8).

The limitations of voice and whisper tests must be borne in mind. They are approximations. Voices vary in clarity and pitch. Nevertheless, these tests are of great value, and should always be carried out before proceeding to tuning fork tests or audiometry.

TUNING FORK TESTS

Before considering the tuning fork tests it is necessary to have a basic conception of the classification of the different types of deafness. Almost every form of deafness (and there are many) may be classified under one of three headings:

Conductive deafness.
Sensorineural deafness.
Mixed conductive and sensorineural.

Conductive deafness (Fig. 10). There is some obstruction, defect or lesion of the external meatus, tympanic membrane, middle ear cavity or ossicles which interferes with the normal passage of air-borne sounds to the cochlea (e.g. wax, perforations, middle ear disease, otosclerosis).

Sensorineural deafness (Fig. 11). There is some defect of the cochlea or auditory nerve whereby nervous impulses from cochlea to brain are attenuated (e.g. Menière's disease, senile deafness, VIIIth nerve tumour).

Mixed deafness. Conductive and sensorineural factors are both present in the same ear.

Explanatory note. Otologists may refer to one patient as having 'good bone-conduction', or to another as having 'poor bone-conduction'. These terms are frequently misunderstood by students, who infer that the skull

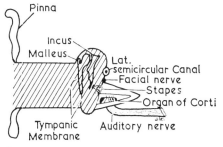

Fig. 10. Conductive deafness is caused by an abnormality of the external or middle ear (shaded).

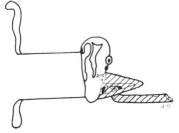

Fig. 11. Sensorineural deafness is caused by an abnormality of the inner ear or auditory nerve (shaded).

of the first patient conducts sound well, and the skull of the second patient conducts sound poorly. This is an understandable misconception.

'Good bone-conduction', or, more correctly, good hearing by bone-conduction, implies a cochlea and auditory nerve which are functioning well. Conversely, 'poor bone-conduction', or, more correctly, poor hearing by bone conduction, implies defective function of cochlea or auditory nerve, in other words—sensorineural deafness.

Rinne's test

The fork—a heavy 512 c.p.s. (cycles per second)—is struck and held close to the meatus until the patient signals that it can no longer be heard. Immediately its base is applied firmly to the mastoid process.

If, then, the patient cannot hear it, he has a normal or positive Rinne, sound being heard better by air-conduction than by bone-conduction. (AC > BC). Deduction. If deafness is present, deafness is sensorineural.

If, on the other hand, the patient can still hear the fork by bone-conduction, he has a negative Rinne. (BC > AC). Deduction. Deafness is conductive.

It will be seen that Rinne's test depends on the fact that more sound reaches the cochlea if it has passed through the magnifying mechanism of the normal middle ear than if it has passed straight through the bone to the cochlea without magnification.

False negative Rinne. Another trap for the unguarded. A patient with severe unilateral perceptive deafness may appear to hear better by BC than AC in the deaf ear. He is, in fact, hearing the bone-conducted sound 'across the way' in his good cochlea (Fig. 14).

If you suspect a false negative Rinne, carry out the test again with the

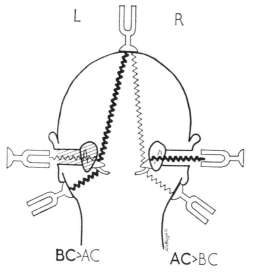

L R

BC>AC AC>BC

Fig. 12. Conductive deafness in the left ear. The left Rinne is negative, and in Weber's test, sound is referred to the left side.

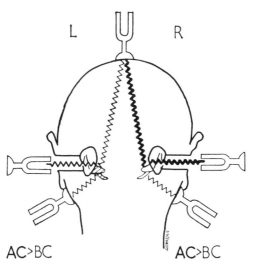

L R

AC>BC AC>BC

Fig. 13. Sensorineural deafness in the left ear. The left Rinne is positive and in Weber's test, sound is referred to the right side.

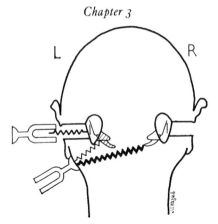

Fig. 14. False negative Rinne. Severe sensorineural deafness left. It appears that sound is heard on the left side better by bone than by air conduction. It is, in fact, being 'picked-up' in the right cochlea.

better ear masked by Bárány's noise apparatus. Little or nothing will be heard by the deaf ear either by air or bone.

Weber's test (Often unreliable)

The base of the fork is held on the vertex, and the patient is asked in which ear he seems to be hearing the sound.

In conductive deafness sound is referred to the deafer ear.

In sensorineural deafness sound is referred to the better ear.

How can sound be referred to a deafer ear? Because if the deafness is of conductive type, the cochlea on that side will be undisturbed by ambient noise (extraneous sounds in the room), and 'is able to concentrate' on the sound arriving by bone conduction. On the other side of the head the normal middle ear mechanism amplifies extraneous sounds which occupy the attention of its cochlea.

Absolute bone conduction

In this test a comparison is made between the perceptive mechanism of the patient and that of the examiner. With the ear under test occluded by pressure on the tragus, the base of the fork is applied to the mastoid process, and the patient signals as soon as the sound disappears. The examiner, with one of his own ears occluded, immediately applies the base of the fork to his own mastoid, and if he can still hear the note it may be deduced that the patient has some degree of sensorineural deafness.

If the examiner is himself afflicted with sensorineural deafness, he will fail to diagnose this condition in his patient, and is advised to abandon the test!

AUDIOMETRY

The audiometer is an electronic instrument capable of generating pure tones ranging from 125 c.p.s. to about 12,000 c.p.s. (Fig. 15).

The operator, by manipulating a control, chooses a tone, which is fed into the patient's ear by means of a headphone. By operating another control the volume is increased until the patient signals that he can just

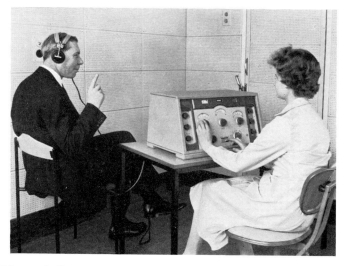

Fig. 15. Audiometry. The patient is signalling that he can hear a test tone.

hear the note emitted. The volume and frequency readings are now recorded, and by making a series of tests the threshold of hearing for each of the test frequencies is charted in the form of an audiogram (Figs. 16, 17, 18). Hearing loss is expressed in decibels, which are logarithmic units of relative intensity.

The patient's hearing acuity by bone-conduction may be tested by substituting for the headphone a small contact receiver applied to the mastoid process.

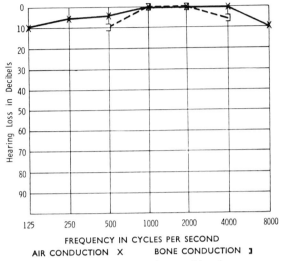

Fig. 16. Audiogram showing good hearing.

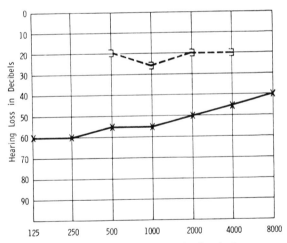

Fig. 17. Audiogram showing conductive deafness.

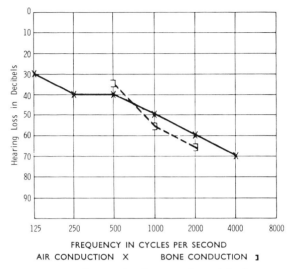

FREQUENCY IN CYCLES PER SECOND
AIR CONDUCTION X   BONE CONDUCTION]

Fig. 18. Audiogram showing sensorineural deafness.

ADVANCED AUDIOLOGY

1 Speech audiometry.
2 Békésy audiometry.
3 Impedance audiometry.
4 Electric response audiometry.
5 Electrocochleography.

Speech audiometry is employed to measure the intelligibility of the spoken word in the patient being tested. The patient listens to recorded test words given at varying sound pressures and a graph can be plotted showing his 'score' at different sound intensities. It is thus possible to show whether he has *loudness recruitment*—that particular malfunction of the cochlea whereby hearing acuity falls off and discomfort increases *disproportionately* as the sound pressure rises.

Békésy audiometry is carried out using instead of the conventional pure-tone audiometer, a more elaborate motorized instrument in which the patient depresses or releases a button according to whether he hears or ceases to hear a test tone. The instrument is thus able to produce a trace from which may be deduced not only the threshold of hearing but the degree of recruitment at any particular frequency. It is a valuable aid to diagnosis, and one of the means of helping in the important distinction of hearing loss due to end-organ disorder and that caused by a lesion of the eighth nerve, e.g. acoustic neuroma.

Impedance audiometry is perhaps likely to be encountered by the house surgeon more frequently than the other advanced techniques. It is the measurement of the impedance of the tympanic membrane and, briefly, this is achieved by feeding sound into the external meatus and measuring the amount of reflected sound with varying air pressure in the meatus.

Impedance audiometry is now routinely employed for **tympanometry** in connection with conditions of the middle ear, e.g. secretory otitis, but it is also used to measure the **acoustic reflex** whereby sound fed into *either* ear at a high level above threshold induces contraction of *both* stapedius muscles, thus altering the impedance of the tympanic membrane. By this means additional information is obtained relating to numerous conditions as varied as facial nerve paralysis and malingering.

Electric response audiometry is a collective term for various methods whereby electrical potentials can be evoked by sound (usually a series of clicks), applied to the ear. Thus cochlear, brainstem and cortical responses may be recorded and are of great value in pin-pointing the site of a lesion in the long and complex auditory pathway.

The methods are elaborate and require the use of averaging devices owing to the huge amount of electrical noise in the body. However, as these tests are objective (unlike routine pure-tone or speech audiometry) they may be applied to non-cooperative patients such as very young children or malingerers.

Special mention should be made of electrocochleography, sometimes referred to as E Coch G, which is available in most centres. A needle electrode is inserted through the tympanic membrane under local analgesia or general anaesthetic, and placed on the promontory. Clicks are then fed into the ear under test and the resulting electric potentials analysed and recorded in graphic form.

Note. The foregoing section is but a perfunctory account of a huge subject and the interested reader can do no better than study the excellent narrative and diagrams given by Graham & Beazley in *Recent Advances in Otolaryngology*. (See my Chapter 48, 'Further Reading and Higher Qualifications'.)

CHAPTER 4
CONDITIONS OF THE AURICLE (PINNA)

CONGENITAL

Protruding ears. Sometimes known as 'bat's' ears. These outstanding auricles are very unsightly, and if uncorrected may cause their owner to be the butt of much ragging in childhood. Surgery should be carried out ideally between the ages of **four years** and **six years,** and consists basically of the excision of an area of post-auricular skin, together with a little auricular cartilage (Fig. 19). The operation is not so simple as might appear at first sight, but requires skill and experience in order to achieve equal success on the two sides as in the case of cosmetic operations on other paired structures.

Accessory auricle. These small tags or nodules are sometimes seen on the cheek between the angle of the mouth and the tragus (Fig. 20).

Fistula auris. A small blind pit seen quite commonly anterior to the

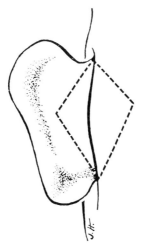

Fig. 19. A protruding ear. The broken line indicates (approx.) the area of soft tissue removed.

17

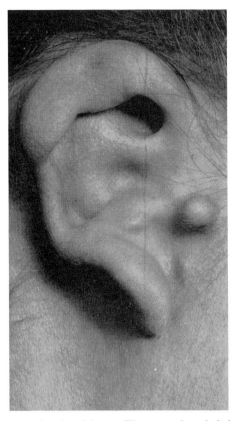

Fig. 20. Congenital deformity of the ear. The meatus is occluded, the helix is incomplete and an accessory auricle is present.

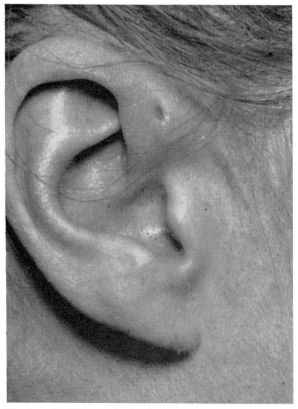

Fig. 21. Fistula auris. (The opening is often nearer the tragus than in this case.)

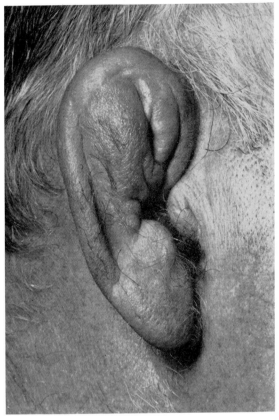

Fig. 22. Haematoma auris—needs careful treatment. A cauliflower ear may ensue.

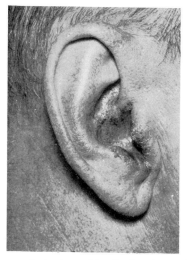

Fig. 23. Acute dermatitis affecting the concha.

tragus. Sometimes bilateral, it results from incomplete fusion of the auricular tubercles. Seldom calls for treatment, but may become infected, when incision or excision is indicated (Fig. 21).

TRAUMA

Haematoma. (Haematoma auris, Othaematoma.) This may follow a blow on the ear, and is common in boxers. It is also seen in Rugby football players as a result of trauma received in the scrum (Fig. 22).

Bleeding takes place between the cartilage and its covering layers of perichondrium. The whole auricle may become ballooned into a bluish, shapeless mass. If untreated, the cartilage necroses, and the auricle becomes an ugly, shrivelled appendage—cauliflower ear.

Treatment consists of aspiration of the clot, and sometimes free incision with compression by bandages or moulded splints in an endeavour to approximate the cartilage and its blood supply—the perichondrium.

INFECTION

Acute dermatitis of the auricle may occur as an extension of the meatal infection in otitis externa, and not infrequently follows the use of

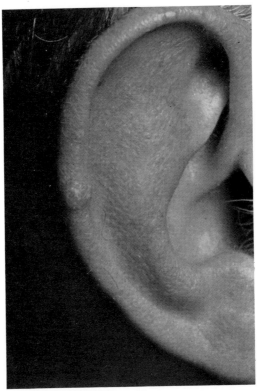

Fig. 24. Chondrodermatitis chronicis helicis. (Dr. P. D. Samman's case.)

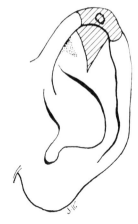

Fig. 25. Epithelioma of the auricle, showing the V-shaped area of excision.

local antibiotics. The oedematous, red auricle desquamates, with the production of copious serous fluid—'weeping eczema' (Fig. 23).

Treatment

1 The otitis externa should be adequately treated (q.v.).
2 The auricle may be coated with a cream of zinc and 2 per cent ichthammol or fluocinolone acetonide cream (Synalar) or betamethasone cream (Betnovate).
3 Bed rest with sedation may hasten improvement and cure in very severe cases.

Perichondritis sometimes follows a haematoma or, very rarely, mastoidectomy. A cauliflower ear is likely to result, and treatment consists of administering the appropriate antibiotic. Incision may be necessary.

Chondrodermatitis chronicis helicis occurs most commonly in elderly males. It is manifested by a nodular and *exquisitely tender* swelling of the helix. It may be ulcerated and its appearance may resemble a neoplasm. Treatment consists of excision of the small mass.

TUMOURS
Epithelioma
Rodent ulcer

These tumours usually occur on the upper edge of the auricle. Either

Chapter 4

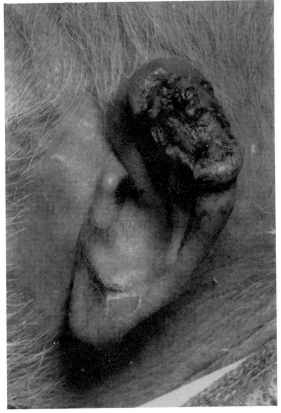

Fig. 26. Epithelioma of the auricle.

tumour is often successfully treated in its earliest stage by a wide V-shaped excision (Fig. 25), but a more advanced tumour with spread to the scalp or (as in the case of Fig. 26), lymph node involvement calls for more radical treatment.

CHAPTER 5
CONDITIONS OF THE EXTERNAL
AUDITORY MEATUS

CONGENITAL

Stenosis of the external auditory meatus. The meatus may be a shallow blind pit. Careful radiological and audiological investigation is called for in order to assess the degree of development of the middle and inner ears.

In **bilateral** cases treatment should be undertaken **early,** and every endeavour must be made by plastic or fenestration techniques to open the pathway of sound to the inner ear.

In **unilateral** cases with good hearing in the contralateral ear treatment may be **delayed.**

FOREIGN BODY

Inanimate foreign bodies. Beads, pips and other objects are sometimes introduced into the external auditory meatus by small children.

Several important points arise:

1 The chief danger lies in clumsy attempts at removal by unskilled persons (who may rupture the tympanic membrane). No attempt to remove a foreign body should be made unless some skill as an aurist has been acquired.

2 If the child is in any way uncooperative it is advisable to resort to general anaesthesia.

3 It is useless to attempt to remove small round objects, such as ball-bearings, with aural forceps. A wax-hook or curette is gently inserted beyond the foreign body.

Insects. The most likely visitor is the common fly, which causes its host appalling irritation with its flapping wings. Peace is quickly restored by dropping olive oil into the ear, and the corpse may then be removed by syringing.

WAX

Wax, or cerumen, is the normal secretion of the ceruminous glands situated in the outer part of the external meatus. There is considerable individual variation in the quantity and quality of wax secreted, most persons forming a small amount of soft wax, which, unnoticed, works its way out of their auditory canals throughout their lifetime.

Wax may, however, be troublesome, and if produced in large quantities, or if unduly hard, it may form an impacted mass, causing deafness and sometimes irritation of the meatal skin.

Ear-syringing, the usual method of removing wax, is an operation which almost any doctor or nurse is expected to carry out with skill, and which the general practitioner should perform with a flawless technique (Fig. 27). Attention must be paid to the following points:

1   History. Has the patient had a discharging ear? If any possibility of a dry perforation, do not syringe.

2   Inspection. If wax seems very hard always soften over a period of one week by using warm olive oil drops nightly. In the case of exceedingly stubborn wax the patient may be advised to use sodium bicarbonate

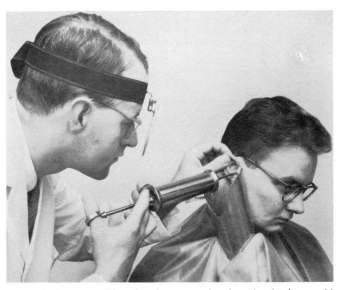

Fig. 27. Syringing an ear. Note that the surgeon is using a head-mirror and is drawing the auricle upwards and backwards in order to 'straighten' the external meatus.

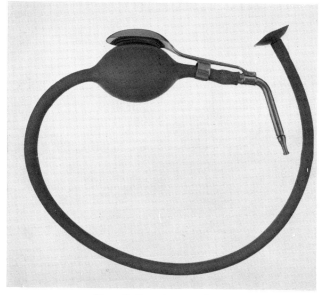

Fig. 28. Bacon's ear syringe.

eardrops (B.P.C.), and there are on the market several 'quick-acting' ceruminolytic agents. Occasionally a patient reacts badly to the use of the latter and develops otitis externa. They should certainly not be employed in the case of a patient who is known to suffer from recurrent infections of the meatal canal.

3   Towels. Protect patient well with towels and mackintoshes. He will not be amused by having his shirt soaked.

4   Lighting. Use a head-mirror or lamp.

5   Solution. Sodium bicarbonate, 4–5 grammes to 500 ml, or normal saline, are ideal. Tap-water is satisfactory.

6   Temperature. This is vital. It should be 38° C (100° F). Any departure of more than a few degrees may precipitate patient on floor with vertigo.

7   Syringe. A metal syringe is considered by some to be the most easily controlled, but others prefer rubber syringes of the Bacon type. In any case make sure that the nozzle is firmly attached to the syringe and is prevented from entering too far into the external meatus. Tympanic membranes have been ruptured by a deeply penetrating nozzle.

8   Direction. Direct stream of solution along roof of auditory canal (Fig. 29).

9   Inspection. After removal of wax, inspect thoroughly to make sure

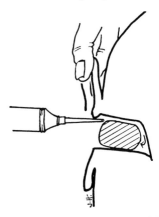

Fig. 29. Direct the stream of solution along the roof of the external auditory meatus.

none remains. This advice might seem superfluous, but is frequently ignored.

10   Drying. Mop any excess solution from meatal canal. Stagnation predisposes to otitis externa.

Students often enquire 'Is it possible to rupture the ear drum with a powerful jet of fluid by exerting too much pressure on the bulb or plunger of the ear syringe?' This accident is extremely unlikely to take place if the tympanic membrane is normal, but it certainly may occur if part of the membrane is scarred.

OTITIS EXTERNA

Otitis externa is a diffuse inflammation of the skin lining the external auditory meatus. It may be bacterial or mycotic (otomycosis), and is characterized by irritation, desquamation, scanty discharge, and tendency to relapse. The treatment is simple, but success is absolutely dependent upon patience, care, and meticulous attention to detail.

Causes

Otitis externa has a predilection for certain persons. Some individuals, after washing or bathing, may allow water to remain in the ears with impunity, but in others, and particularly in those with a tendency to eczema, this oversight invites trouble. Those who frequent crowded swimming baths, and refrain from drying their ears, or traumatize them with the screwed-up corner of a dirty towel, are particularly prone.

Scratching with the finger nails inflicts further trauma and introduces new organisms. A vicious circle is set up.

Otitis externa is frequently seen in Europeans visiting the tropics, where increased sweat secretion, dust and bathing in infected water are predisposing factors.

Ear-syringing is sometimes responsible, particularly if any trauma has been inflicted, or if a remnant of moist wax is overlooked.

Pathology

A mixed infection of varying organisms is not infrequent, the most commonly found types being:

Staph. pyogenes
Ps. pyocyanea
Diphtheroids
Proteus vulgaris
Esch. coli
Str. faecalis
Aspergillus niger
Candida albicans.

Symptoms

Irritation.
Discharge (scanty).
Pain (usually moderate, sometimes severe, increased by jaw movement).
Deafness.

Signs

Tenderness (particularly on compression of the tragus).
Moist debris, the removal of which reveals:

Red desquamated meatal walls.
Oedema of the meatal skin.

Management

Investigation into the bacteriology is made by submitting an aural swab for culture and it is prudent to mention in your request the possibi-

Fig. 30. Jobson Horne wool carrier. An invaluable instrument.

lity of fungal contamination. Cases of otomycosis are sometimes particularly resistant to treatment and must be treated with the most appropriate medicaments.

Aural toilet with the removal of every particle of debris is the cornerstone of treatment. The instrument of choice is the Jobson Horne wool carrier dressed with fluffed-out cotton wool (Fig. 30). The meatus is gradually cleared by a gentle rotatory mopping action, and as soon as the wool is soiled it is discarded and replaced. The antero-inferior meatal recess must receive special attention. It commonly acts as a sump for debris and organisms.

Dressings. Following cleansing, a length of half-inch ribbon gauze, or a small spill of cotton wool soaked in one of the following medicaments, should be inserted into the meatus with aural dressing forceps, and left for twenty-four hours. (Fig. 31). The dressing should be renewed daily until the appearance of the meatal skin has returned to normal.

Many different medicaments have been used in the treatment of otitis externa, some of the most useful being as follows:
1·5 per cent hydrocortisone with neomycin sulphate (dressings);
8 per cent aluminium acetate (dressings);
10 per cent ichthammol in glycerine (dressings).

In cases of otomycosis the following applications are particularly useful:
Amphotericin B, 3 per cent aqueous solution (Fungilin) dressings.
Gentian violet, 1 per cent aqueous solution (painted on meatal walls).
Powder containing 0·4 per cent hydrargaphen (Penotrane) insufflated in
    meatus.

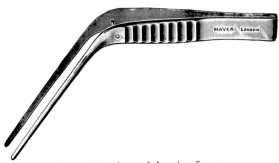

Fig. 31. Keen's aural dressing forceps.

Salicylic acid, 2 per cent in 70 per cent alcohol (used as drops).

General treatment with analgesics, sedatives, or systemic antibiotics is necessary in a few cases, and very heavy sedation, with bed rest, may have to be resorted to in any severe case with an associated anxiety state.

Advice to the patient, if implemented, lessens the chance of recurrence:

1 Keep water out of the ears.
2 Don't scratch the ears.

Causes of failure in effecting a cure

The chief cause of failure in the treatment of otitis externa is the omission of *thorough aural cleansing.* In fact many cases could be cured by cleansing alone and without resorting to the use of dressings, drops, powders and paints. How can drops effect a cure when they are poured day after day into meatal canals stuffed with debris?

The use of certain preparations locally may serve to make matters worse by setting up an eczematous reaction. Penicillin and chloramphenicol are noted for their activity in this sphere and even neomycin can cause a severe dermatitis if applied for long periods.

Another cause of failure is underlying seborrhoeic dermatitis for which an expert opinion should be sought. Finally, it must be mentioned that poor results are usually obtained in the unhygienic and uncooperative patient, who scratches and rubs his ears ceaselessly, thereby continually reinfecting them.

FURUNCULOSIS

Boils are due to infection of the hair follicles of the meatus. The following points are noteworthy:

1 Limited to the outer part of the meatus.
2 Caused by staphylococcus.
3 Often occur in patients who are 'run-down' or subject to infections (e.g. diabetics).
4 Sometimes bilateral.

Symptoms

Pain (as incapacitating as severe toothache. Made worse by jaw movements.)

Deafness.

Signs

Marked tenderness on compression of tragus.
Severe pain elicited by moving auricle.
One or more boils present in outer part of meatus, partially or wholly obliterating the lumen.

Treatment

A narrow spill of wool soaked in 10 per cent ichthammol in glycerine should be gently inserted into the meatus and replaced once or twice daily.

Analgesics are usually indicated, and the patient is not fit for work.

Local heat in the form of radiant heat, electric-pad or short-wave diathermy is helpful.

In some cases systemic antibiotics may be necessary.

In recurrent cases:

1 Exclude predisposing causes (diabetes, malnutrition, etc.);
2 Try staphylococcal vaccine (autogenous or stock).

EXOSTOSES

Exostoses or small osteomata of the external auditory meatus are fairly common and usually bilateral. There is no doubt that they are the result of prolonged exposure to cold water, and they are frequently possessed by those hardy characters who take pleasure in swimming, diving and other aquatic sports, even under the most inclement climatic conditions.

There may be two or three of the little tumours arising in each bony meatus. They are sessile, hard, smooth, covered with very thin skin and when gently probed are often exquisitely sensitive. Their rate of growth is extremely slow, and they may give rise to no symptoms, but if wax or debris accumulates between the tympanic membrane and the exostoses, its removal may tax the patience of the most skilled manipulator. In such cases, where recurrent trouble is encountered, surgical removal of the exostoses may be indicated and is carried out with the aid of operating microscope and dental burr.

MALIGNANT DISEASE

This commences as a small epitheliomatous ulcer or friable mass. It is fortunately rare, occurring more commonly in the elderly. It is a relentless and terrible affliction. There are two important early symptoms:

Pain becoming intractable and intolerable.

Bloodstained discharge from the ear.

Spread is by local extension in the middle ear, facial nerve and temporomandibular joint, and by lymphatics to the upper cervical nodes.

X-rays may show bony loss, and the diagnosis is confirmed by biopsy.

Treatment is by radiotherapy or radical surgery, or a combination of the two. The outlook is poor.

CHAPTER 6
INJURY OF THE
TYMPANIC MEMBRANE

DIVERSE circumstances may be responsible for injury or rupture of the tympanic membrane, and the early treatment of such injury is of great importance. Ignorance may prove disastrous.

Causes

Direct trauma. Attempts to remove wax or foreign bodies by the unskilled.

Blast, gunfire, fireworks, rapid descent in aircraft, slap on the ear.

Fracture—of the temporal bone.

Symptoms

Pain. (Acute at the moment of rupture. Usually transient.)

Deafness.

Tinnitus.

Vertigo. (Rarely.)

Signs

Bleeding from the ear. (Sometimes.)

Bloodclot in the meatus.

A tear in the tympanic membrane.

Treatment

Do NOT *clean out the ear or remove the clot.*

Do NOT *put in drops.*

Do NOT *syringe.*

Do NOT *interfere.*

Watch the ear daily, and in most cases the edges of the tear will unite rapidly. If there are any signs of infection supervening, e.g. discharge, give systemic antibiotics.

CHAPTER 7
ACUTE OTITIS MEDIA

ACUTE bacterial inflammation of the middle ear cavity is a common condition and frequently bilateral. It occurs most often in children, and it is of the utmost importance to the community that medical practitioners should be well acquainted with its pathology, treatment and complications. Infection usually arrives via the Eustachian tube (Fig. 32), but occasionally by other routes.

CAUSES

More common
- Acute tonsillitis
- Common cold
- Influenza
- Coryza of measles, scarlet fever, whooping cough, etc.

Less common
- Sinusitis
- Tonsillectomy
- Diving
- Trauma of tympanic membrane (blast, f.b., slap, etc)
- Otitic barotrauma (sudden descent in aircraft)
- Fracture of temporal bone
- Infantile gastroenteritis
- Post-nasal plug

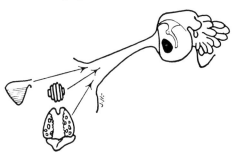

Fig. 32. The most common sources of the infection in acute otitis media— tonsils, adenoids and sinuses.

PATHOLOGY

There is usually a pure infection of:

Haemolytic streptococcus or
Pneumococcus or
Staphylococcus.

Acute otitis media is an infection of the mucous membrane lining the whole of the middle ear cleft—Eustachian tube, tympatic cavity, attic, aditus, mastoid antrum, mastoid cells. (What then is acute mastoiditis? The bony necrosis of the cells owing to faulty drainage and/or virulent infection.)

The sequence of events in acute otitis media is as follows:

1   Organisms invade the mucous membrane, causing inflammation, with hyperaemia (red drum), oedema and serous (later purulent) exudate.
2   Oedema closes escape route down Eustachian tube (Fig. 33).
3   Pressure increases in tympanic cavity bulging tympanic membrane.
4   T.M. ruptures.
5   Discharge continues to escape through perforation until infection resolves.

SYMPTOMS

Earache. This is usually severe and throbbing. A young child may cry and scream for hours until it falls into a fitful sleep in a state of exhaustion.

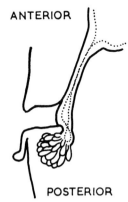

ANTERIOR

POSTERIOR

Fig. 33. Diagrammatic transverse section to show the middle ear cleft (left). The mucosal lining of the Eustachian tube has become oedematous as a result of infection.

Deafness is of conductive type and is sometimes accompanied by tinnitus. In an adult the deafness or tinnitus may be the first complaint.

SIGNS

Pyrexia. The child is flushed. Temperature may be as high as 39·4° C.

Tenderness. There is usually some tenderness on pressure over the mastoid antrum.

The tympanic membrane varies in appearance according to the stage of the infection:

1   Loses its lustre. Cone of light absent.
2   Pink. Vessels have made appearance down handle of malleus and around periphery.
3   Red and full. Handle of malleus is vertical.
4   Bulging. Plum colour. Landmarks lost. Outer layer of T.M. may desquamate causing slight bloodstained serous discharge.
5   Perforation.

Discharge is usually profuse and mucoid at first. May be pulsating. Later thick and yellow.

X-rays usually show some opacity of the mastoid cells.

TREATMENT

The treatment depends on the stage reached by the infection. The following stages may be considered:

1   Early.
2   Bulging.
3   Discharging.

1   Early

Antibiotics. Penicillin. Two large doses by injection, followed by oral preparation for at least 5 days. In the absence of a rapid response change to wide-spectrum antibiotic.

Analgesics. In children, aspirin or Nepenthe. In adults, codeine, Physeptone, pethidine.

Nasal vasconstrictors. One-half per cent ephedrine in normal saline nasal drops q.d.s.

Analgesic ear-drops are sometimes advised, but tend to obscure the tympanic membrane, and may be mistaken for discharge.

Attention to coexistent infection, e.g. sinusitis, tonsillitis, etc.

2   Bulging

Myringotomy is indicated when *bulging* of the tympanic membrane or *pain* persist in spite of antibiotic therapy, though it seldom has to be performed these days. Under general anaesthesia, and with aseptic precautions, the tympanic membrane is incised posterior to the handle of the

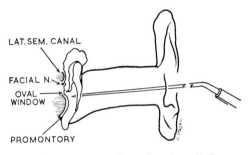

LAT. SEM. CANAL

FACIAL N.

OVAL WINDOW

PROMONTORY

Fig. 34. Myringotomy. Coronal section of left ear.

malleus (Figs. 34 and 35). In the bad old days the performance of this operation was often relegated to inexperienced persons, but a glance at the nature and proximity of the anatomical relations (Figs. 4 and 34) will amply demonstrate the folly of that custom. It is essential not to plunge the myringotome deeply through the tympanic membrane—1 *millimetre should suffice*—and the presence, close by, of such structures as the incudo-stapedial joint, facial nerve, etc., must be borne in mind.

If possible the surgeon should have acquired some experience of aural work using a binocular loupe or operating microscope.

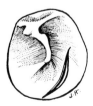

Fig. 35. Myringotomy. The extent of the incision.

As the myringotome pierces the tympanic membrane pus escapes and must be examined bacteriologically.

Antibiotics. Myringotomy having been performed it is now possible to pin-point the organism and give the appropriate antibiotic.

Aural toilet is now necessary. The ear should be dry-mopped with cotton wool two or three times daily. Gentle irrigation with normal saline at 38° C (100° F), followed by dry mopping is sometimes found more efficacious. Ear-drops are unnecessary.

3 Discharging

Frequently, medical attention is not sought until the tympanic membrane has ruptured, and discharge commenced. In these circumstances, attention has to be paid to the administration of:

Appropriate antibiotic.

Regular aural toilet.

FURTHER MANAGEMENT

If treatment has been administered early and antibiotics have been given in adequate dosage and for sufficient time, most cases of acute otitis media resolve, and hearing returns to normal.

Occasionally, discharge continues, or deafness persists, or, worse still, the symptoms and signs of acute mastoiditis, or intracranial complications appear. (The latter are dealt with in a separate section.)

In the event of continued discharge or deafness:

1 Suspect the nose and nasopharynx—infection may be present.
2 Suspect the choice of antibiotic.
3 Suspect low-grade infection in middle ear and mastoid cells.

SUMMARY OF TREATMENT

1 Antibiotics.
2 Analgesics.
3 Myringotomy (under certain circumstances).
4 Nasal vasoconstrictors.
5 Aural toilet, if any discharge.
6 Careful observation.
7 Search for sepsis, if recovery incomplete.

CHAPTER 8
CHRONIC OTITIS MEDIA

IN some cases of acute otitis media, the pain and temperature subside, but the infection persists, the perforation remains unhealed, and discharge continues. A mixed infection by several different types of organism is now present, and as the damage to the middle ear increases, so does the degree of conductive deafness.

This is chronic (suppurative) otitis media (C.S.O.M.). The predisposing causes are as follows:

1 The acute infection was not treated early.
2 Dosage of antibiotics was inadequate.
3 Antibiotics were discontinued too soon.
4 Nasal or pharyngeal sepsis is present.
5 Lowered resistance (e.g. malnutrition, anaemia) is present.
6 The infection is particularly virulent.

There are two main types of chronic otitis media—the **mucosal type** and the **bony type,** the latter being manifest either as generalized mastoid disease or as attic disease.

MUCOSAL TYPE OF INFECTION

In these cases there is often underlying nasal or pharyngeal sepsis, e.g. chronic infection of the tonsils or sinuses, or adenoidal hypertrophy.

The discharge is definitely mucoid, and the perforation is in the central part of the pars tensa (Fig. 36).

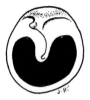

Fig. 36. A large central perforation as seen in the mucosal type of C.S.O.M.

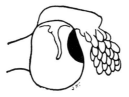

Fig. 37. A postero-superior marginal perforation as seen in the bony type of C.S.O.M.

Serious complications are rare, but if the disease is allowed to progress the perforation will become larger and deafness will increase.

The infection may be quiescent from time to time, when examination will reveal a dry perforation or a perforation which has become replaced by thin scar tissue.

BONY TYPE OF INFECTION

The bone affected by disease comprises the tympanic ring, the ossicles, the mastoid air cells and to some extent the bony walls of the tympanic cavity, attic, aditus and antrum. The perforation is marginal and posterior, and the discharge is purulent and sometimes evil-smelling (Fig. 37).

In the so-called *attic-disease*, infection is limited to the head of the malleus, the incus, and the attic. The perforation is in the pars flaccida (Schrapnell's membrane) (Fig. 38).

Serious complications much more commonly result from bony disease of the mastoid and attic than from mucosal infection of the middle ear, and are sometimes heralded by an acute exacerbation of the infection with pain and pyrexia.

In addition to the perforation, which increases in size eventually de-

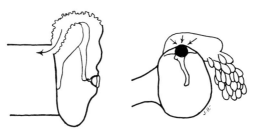

Fig. 38. A perforation in Schrapnell's membrane in the 'attic' type of C.S.O.M.

stroying the whole tympanic membrane, other features are sometimes present:

1 Granulations. Sessile. Bright red. Bleed when touched.

2 Aural polypi. Pedunculated granulations. One polypus may fill the meatus and present at the concha.

3 Cholesteatoma. This is an accumulation of keratotic debris which first forms in a so-called 'retraction pocket' in close relationship to the tympanic annulus. Eventually it invades the attic region and destroys ossicles and surrounding bone by pressure. It may in fact cause an enormous cavity invading the internal ear and middle and posterior cranial fossae, thus opening up pathways for the spread of infection to the meninges and brain. In appearance a cholesteatomatous deposit is usually a flaky and dead-white in colour and may smell of cats!

4 X-ray changes include loss of outline of the mastoid cells, opacity suggesting sclerosis, and, in the case of a cholesteatomatous deposit of any size—a translucent area suggesting cavitation.

5 Fistula sign. Increase of pressure in external auditory meatus causes vertigo and sometimes nystagmus, demonstrating fistula between middle ear and labyrinth (Fig. 39).

Treatment

Conservative treatment in chronic otitis media consists of (1) attention to the general state of health, (2) the eradication of sepsis from the upper respiratory tract, e.g. tonsillectomy or sinus drainage if necessary, and (3) local aural toilet.

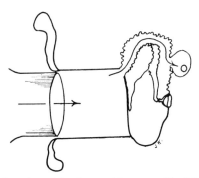

Fig. 39. Fistula in lateral semicircular canal in a case of 'attic' disease. The fistula sign is positive.

The latter is of great importance and should be carried out two or three times daily, ideally by skilled personnel using a Jobson Horne wool carrier (Fig. 30). Obviously such attention can only be obtained in highly organized clinics but the intelligent patient can often be taught to mop the ear with orange sticks dressed with fluffed-out cotton wool or simply with wool spills.

After the ear has been cleaned drops may be instilled. It is certainly popular practice to use antibiotic solutions for this purpose but they carry a risk of skin sensitization and a more remote risk of ototoxicity. The time-honoured **25 or 50 per cent spirit** ear-drops are hard to beat but patients using them should always be warned in advance that they may 'sting'.

When large barely-moist perforations are present **1 per cent iodine in boric acid powder** may be insufflated occasionally and often renders the ear completely dry.

Operative treatment in chronic otitis media embraces many techniques, and is indicated *when the disease progresses in spite of conservation treatment*.

1   **Suction clearance** is carried out under the microscope in many early cases of chronic otitis media. With the aid of suitable suction apparatus cholesteatoma and granulation tissue are removed via the perforation and any aural polypi can also be dealt with. A proportion of cases respond admirably to this simple form of treatment and a dry ear may result.

2   **Cortical mastoidectomy** is sometimes adequate in early cases of chronic otitis media. It is described under acute mastoiditis, for which it is more commonly indicated.

3   **Radical mastoidectomy** may be required when disease has progressed far, with severe deafness and the possibility of intracranial complication. Via an endaural or postaural incision the surgeon exenterates the mastoid cells and clears all diseased tissue from the antrum, aditus, attic and tympanic cavity, together with any remains of tympanic membrane and ossicles, with the exception of the footplate of the stapes. The object is to create one large cavity draining freely into an enlarged external auditory meatus. Discharge may, in some cases, persist, but the patient is safe, though usually very deaf.

4   **Epitympanic mastoidectomy** is sometimes employed in cases of attic disease with good hearing. Again, the mastoid cells, antrum, aditus and attic are cleared of diseased tissue but every effort is made to retain the integrity of the pars tensa and ossicular chain, preserving the hearing.

5   **Tympanoplasty.** With increasing efforts to preserve function the

Chapter 8

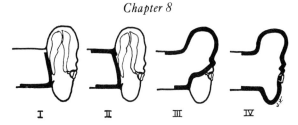

Fig. 40. Tympanoplasty—types I–IV. Vein or fascia graft (thick lines) are used in an attempt to reconstruct the sound-conducting mechanism after varying degrees of damage.

conventional forms of mastoidectomy are performed less frequently and where possible the techniques of tympanoplasty are applied. In these operations all diseased tissue is carefully eradicated and an attempt is made to reconstruct the sound-conducting mechanisms of the middle ear by replacing the tympanic membrane with vein graft or temporal fascia and by utilizing undamaged ossicles.

In the earlier days of tympanoplasty a mastoidectomy-like cavity was often made (Fig. 40). But latterly with the **combined approach tympanoplasty,** a technique demanding the highest degree of surgical skill, the meatal canal wall is preserved intact and the deeper recesses of the tympanum are drained via a posterior tympanotomy or opening *between* the tympanic ring and the descending portion of the facial nerve.

6 Myringoplasty is the term usually applied to the most 'simple' form of tympanoplasty—the closure of a perforation in the tympanic membrane. It is only appropriate in the absence of diseased tissue in the middle ear and better results are obtained in the complete absence of discharge at the time of operation. During the last 25 years numerous tissues have been used as grafts to repair the tympanic membrane, including skin, venous wall, conjunctiva and mucous membrane, but the one tissue which has stood the test of time and, at the time of writing, is almost universally employed is temporalis fascia.

SUMMARY

C.S.O.M.

Deafness
Discharge
Mixed flora
Mucosal type

Mucoid discharge
Central perforation
Sometimes nasal or pharyngeal sepsis
Complications rare
Bony type
Purulent discharge
Posterior marginal or attic perforation
Granulations, polypi or cholesteatoma may be present
Complications are less remote

TREATMENT

Conservative
Eradicate sepsis
Improve health
Local aural toilet
Surgical
Suction clearance
Mastoidectomy (whichever of the three types is most appropriate)
Tympanoplasty if appropriate
Myringoplasty if appropriate

CHAPTER 9
COMPLICATIONS OF
MIDDLE EAR INFECTION

Acute mastoiditis

Meningitis

Extradural abscess

Petrositis

Facial paralysis

Labyrinthitis

Lateral sinus thrombosis

Brain abscess

Subdural abscess

ACUTE MASTOIDITIS

Acute mastoiditis is the result of extension of infection through the

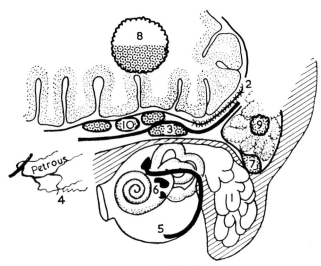

Fig. 41. The complications of middle ear infection.
1 Mastoiditis.
2 Meningitis.
3 Extradural abscess.
4 Petrositis.
5 Facial nerve paralysis.
6 Labyrinthitis.
7 Lateral sinus throm-
bosis.
8 Temporal lobe abscess.
9 Cerebellar abscess.
10 Subdural abscess.

aditus, and may be defined as a suppurative process of the mastoid air-cells associated with bone necrosis and faulty drainage. Factors predisposing to its development are as follows:

Virulent infection.
Low resistance of patient.
Inadequate treatment of the otitis media.
Great cellularity of mastoid.

CLINICAL FEATURES

Symptoms

1 Pain. Persistent and throbbing.
2 Discharge. Usually creamy and profuse.
3 Deafness. Increasing.

Signs

1 Temperature. Remains raised.
2 Pulse. Often disproportionately high.
3 General state. Patient is now obviously ill.
4 Tenderness is marked over mastoid antrum and process.
5 Swelling. Often present over mastoid process. May push auricle forward.
6 Sagging. Of meatal roof near T.M. An important sign.

Investigations

1 White cell count. Usually rising.
2 X-rays. Usually show loss of cell outline (Figs. 42 and 43).

Occasional features of acute mastoiditis are:
1 Sub-periosteal abscess over mastoid process.
2 Bezold's abscess. Pus, tracking down sterno-mastoid sheath, forms abscess in neck.
3 Zygomatic mastoiditis. Swelling over the zygoma results from infection of zygomatic cells.

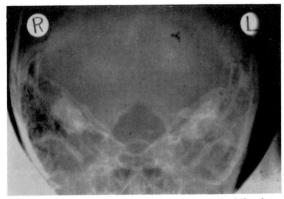

Fig. 42. Acute mastoiditis on the left side. Note the clearly defined mastoid cells on the right in contrast with the general haziness and loss of structure on the left.

TREATMENT

When the diagnosis of acute mastoiditis has been made action must be taken.

1   **Antibiotics.** The appropriate antibiotic should be administered in full dosage.

Choice of antibiotic depends on sensitivity of predominant organism. If sensitivity is not known, penicillin injections are commenced immediately, and sensitivity is determined as soon as possible.

2   **Cortical mastoidectomy** is indicated if the infection does not respond both rapidly and completely.

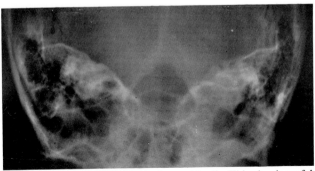

Fig. 43. A Towne's view showing normal mastoid cells. This view is useful in comparing the two sides.

Cortical mastoidectomy (Schwartze operation)

The mastoid process is displayed through a curved post-auricular incision. The cortex is removed by gouges and bone-forceps, or by cutting burs, and all the cells, together with the antrum, are opened. Debris, pus and granulations are removed, with the formation of one large cavity. The scalp-wound is closed, though a small drainage-tube is usually left for a few days. The object of this operation is to drain the mastoid antrum and cells, but to leave untouched the tympanic cavity and membrane, the attic, the ossicles and the external auditory meatus.

Cortical mastoidectomy is an operation requiring skill, experience and much patience. Especial care must be taken in avoiding injury to:

1   The facial nerve.
2   The middle ear mechanism.
3   The lateral sinus.
4   The dura mater.

MENINGITIS

CLINICAL FEATURES

1   Pyrexia.
2   Headache.
3   Neck rigidity.
4   Positive Kernig's sign.
5   Photophobia.
6   C.S.F.
    Often cloudy
    Pressure raised
    Cells raised, polymorphonuclears
    Protein raised
    Chlorides lowered
    Glucose lowered

TREATMENT

1   **Penicillin**—intramuscularly and intrathecally.
2   **Mastoidectomy**—usually performed after the infection has been controlled. The type of operation, i.e. cortical, epitympanic or radical,

depends on the extent of the middle ear and mastoid disease. In some cases, e.g. following otitis media, mastoidectomy may not be necessary.

EXTRADURAL ABSCESS

An abscess forming by direct extension either around the lateral sinus (peri-sinus abscess) or above the tegmen.

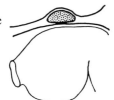

CLINICAL FEATURES

The features of mastoiditis are present and often accentuated. Severe pain is common.

TREATMENT

1 **Antibiotics.**
2 **Mastoidectomy.** Type of operation depends on extent of disease. Abscess is drained via the mastoid cavity.

PETROSITIS

Rare. Infection extends to the apex of the petrous involving the sixth cranial nerve.

CLINICAL FEATURES (Gradenigo's syndrome)

Diplopia due to sixth nerve paresis.
Headache.
Trigeminal pain.
Signs of middle ear infection.

TREATMENT

1 **Antibiotics.**
2 **Mastoidectomy.** Type of operation depends on extent of disease.

FACIAL PARALYSIS

May occur at any stage of middle ear or mastoid infection, acute or chronic.

CLINICAL FEATURES

In the earliest stages the patient may complain of
a slight tendency to dribble from one corner
of the mouth.

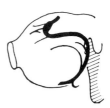

On routine testing the diagnosis becomes obvious.

TREATMENT

1   **Antibiotics.**
2   **Mastoidectomy.** Type of operation depends on extent of disease.

LABYRINTHITIS

Infection may reach the labyrinth via a fistula
in the medial wall of the middle ear. It
occasionally arises in acute otitis media when the
infection is probably blood-borne.

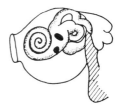

CLINICAL FEATURES

1   Vertigo.
2   Nausea.
3   Vomiting.
4   Nyastagmus.
5   Fistula test, sometimes positive.

The clinical picture varies considerably from one of mild occasional
giddiness, with a positive fistula test—**circumscribed labyrinthis,** to
the overwhelming vertigo of **diffuse purulent labyrinthis.**

TREATMENT

1   **Antibiotics.**
2   **Mastoidectomy.**

The treatment is highly specialized and depends on the type of labyrinthitis. In diffuse serous labyrinthitis associated with acute otitis media,
antibiotics should suffice to control the infection. On the other hand,
radical mastoidectomy would be necessary in a case of cholesteatoma with
fistula and circumscribed labyrinthitis. Occasionally labyrinthectomy is
indicated.

LATERAL SINUS THROMBOSIS

Pus tracks through from the mastoid cells forming
a peri-sinus abscess. Thrombosis takes place in the
lateral sinus, and in an untreated case the
thrombus becomes infected. Ultimately, emboli are
thrown off and cause metastatic abscesses.
Prognosis poor. With early diagnosis and treatment
the prognosis is good.

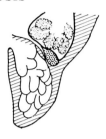

CLINICAL FEATURES

Swinging temperature, e.g. 37° C–40·4° C.
Rigors.
Leucocytosis polymorph.
Positive Tobey-Ayer test—sometimes.
   Compression of contralateral internal jugular vein→rise in C.S.F.
   pressure.
   Compression of ipsilateral internal jugular vein→no rise.
Meningeal signs—sometimes.
Tenderness of ipsilateral internal jugular vein—sometimes.
Positive blood culture—sometimes.
Papilloedema—suggests possible extension to cavernous sinus.
Distant metastatic abscesses—outlook poor.

TREATMENT

1 **Antibiotics.**
2 **Mastoidectomy.**
   Mastoidectomy is essential. In most cases a wide exposure of the sinus
wall is sufficient, but occasionally exploration of the sinus and further
surgery is necessary.

BRAIN ABSCESS

Otogenic brain abscess may occur in the **cerebellum** or the temporal lobe
of the **cerebrum**. The two routes by which infection usually reaches the
brain are as follows:
1 Via bone and meninges, i.e. direct spread; or
2 Via blood vessels, i.e. thrombophlebitis.

A brain abscess may develop with great speed or may gradually develop over a period of months, when certain stages may be recognized.

Invasion—headache, nausea, slight C.S.F. changes.
Latent—transient attacks of headache, etc. Malaise.
Manifest—localizing signs. C.S.F. pressure effects.

GENERAL CLINICAL FEATURES

The symptoms and signs due to invasion and raised intracranial pressure are similar in the case of cerebellar abscess and temporal lobe abscess. They are as follows:

1   Headache, usually on the side of the lesion.
2   Malaise—patient may look toxic.
3   Nausea and vomiting.
4   Pyrexia, irregular, occasional remissions.
5   Papilloedema, may be late.
6   Apathy and drowsiness.
7   Delirium—sometimes.
8   Rigors and convulsions—sometimes.
9   C.S.F.
    Often clear
    Pressure raised
    Cells raised, mononuclears
    Protein raised
    Chlorides normal or lowered
    Glucose normal or lowered

Temporal lobe abscess. Localizing signs.

1   Dysphasia. Nominal type. More common when abscess is on left side. Sometimes.
2   Contralateral upper quadrantic homonymous hemianopia. Sometimes. (Due to involvement of optic radiations.)
3   Paralysis. Contralateral. Face and arm. Rarely leg.
4   Hallucinations of taste and smell. Déja vu. Sometimes.

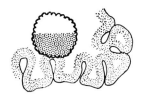

Cerebellar abscess. Localizing signs.

1   Neck stiffness—often.
2   Weakness and loss of tone on same side.
3   Ataxia. Tends to fall to same side.
4   Intention tremor, with past-pointing.
5   Dysdiadokokinesis.
6   Nystagmus—coarse and slow.
7   Vertigo—sometimes.

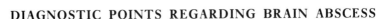

DIAGNOSTIC POINTS REGARDING BRAIN ABSCESS

1   Any patient who has, or has *had*, middle ear infection, and who complains of headache, nausea or malaise, should be suspected of having intracranial suppuration.
2   Any patient who is suffering from otogenic meningitis, labyrinthitis, or lateral sinus thrombosis may also have a brain abscess.
3   Lumbar puncture may be dangerous. (Pressure-cone.)
4   Skilled neurological and neuro-surgical advice should be sought early, and the following techniques may be employed in order to confirm the diagnosis and to locate the abscess:
Air-encephalography.
Angiography.
Brain scan.
Computerized tomography.
Electro-encephalography.
Radio-isotope studies.
5   Finally, it cannot be over-emphasized that the otologist should regard what may appear to be minimal symptoms and signs, with the utmost suspicion *if the patient has had antibiotics* during his illness. So profound may be their *masking* effect and so deluding for the clinician that in general they are best avoided in the treatment of chronic suppurative otitis media, except under conditions of strict control.

Once the abscess has been firmly diagnosed, however, the use of antibiotics must not be delayed.

TREATMENT

Antibiotics.
Tapping through burr holes with replacement by penicillin and thoro-trast (Fig. 44).

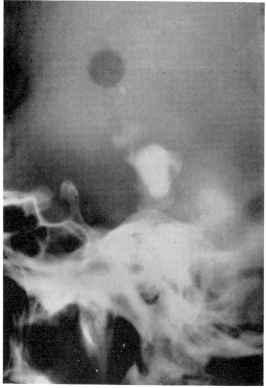

Fig. 44. Lateral view showing burr hole and a temporal lobe abscess outlined by contrast medium.

Excision of the abscess if repeated tapping does not succeed.

Mastoidectomy.

Finally, air-encephalography to exclude any undiscovered abscess or loculus.

NOTE: *If the diagnosis of abscess is in doubt, mastoidectomy is performed first and the patient kept under strict surveillance with a view to burr hole exploration if necessary.*

Prognosis. With antibiotics and modern techniques the prognosis has undergone great improvement, and to-day considerably more than 50 per cent of cases survive. In fact, in one famous neuro-surgical centre the mortality rate has been reduced, in recent years, to the region of 5 per cent. The prognosis is worse for cerebellar than for temporal lobe abscesses.

Untreated, a brain abscess may (1) result in a pressure-cone, (2) rupture into a ventricle, or (3) give rise to spreading encephalitis, in each case with fatal results.

SUBDURAL ABSCESS

Multiple abscesses sometimes occur in the subdural space, the most suggestive clinical feature being the occurrence of focal epileptic fits as a result of cortical involvement.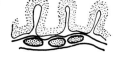

The highly specialized treatment entails drainage through multiple burr holes. Prognosis—poor.

CHAPTER 10
SECRETORY OTITIS MEDIA

SECRETORY otitis media (catarrhal otitis media, glue ear) is a condition of much importance to the practitioner for it is seen with increasing frequency, and failure to recognize it early and treat it energetically may result in permanent deafness.

Causes

1   Nasopharyngeal infections, obstructions (e.g. adenoids) and tumours causing Eustachian insufficiency. This insufficiency is sometimes associated with repeated attacks of acute otitis media and sometimes with the development of an effusion in the middle ear.

2   Otitic barotrauma. This is most commonly seen when landing in an aircraft. Owing to the presence of Eustachian insufficiency air cannot enter the middle ear via the tube. The tympanic membrane is therefore forced inwards and a middle ear effusion often results.

3   It is now considered probable that repeated and inadequate courses of antibiotics for attacks of otitis media may predispose to the formation of a middle ear effusion (secretory otitis media).

Symptoms

Deafness.
Discomfort—'a stuffy feeling' in the ear.
Occasionally, transient pain and tinnitus.

Signs

Fluid in middle ear (Fig. 45).
Yellowish tinge of tympanic membrane (sometimes).
Hair-lines (sometimes).
Tuning forks show conductive deafness.
Impedance curve significantly flattened.

57

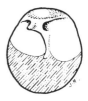

Fig. 45. Secretory otitis. Fluid is present in the
tympanum, and well defined hair-lines are visible.

Treatment

In children

1 **Politzerization.** This is accomplished by means of Politzer's bag, the
nozzle of which is firmly applied to one nostril, the other being compressed. The bag is suddenly squeezed as the child swallows, thus raising
the pressure in the nose and nasopharynx, opening the Eustachian tubes,
and promoting drainage of fluid (Fig. 46). The technique is repeated daily,
and may be carried out by trained nursing staff; it is combined with the use
of nasal vasoconstrictor drops (0·5 per cent ephedrine in normal saline).

Although this conservative method of treatment was often continued
for prolonged periods in the past it is now generally recommended to give
it only a brief trial and in the event of failure to proceed to the surgical
method described below.

2 **Myringotomy and insertion of drain.** This method of treatment
has gained enormous popularity in the last few years. Under a short
general anaesthetic and with the aid of the operating microscope or
binocular loupe a small incision with the myringotome is made in the
inferior part of the tympanic membrane. The serous effusion or 'glue' is
removed by suction, and a Teflon drain or grommet is inserted. These
drainage tubes cause no adverse reaction and may be left *in situ* for long

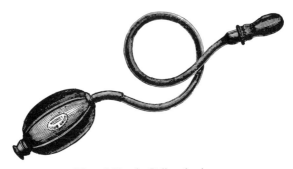

Fig. 46. Bag for Politzerization.

periods or until they are finally extruded. Their most important function is to equalize the air pressures on both sides of the tympanic membrane. If adenoids are present (as they usually are in these cases) they are meticulously removed under the same anaesthetic. Almost all otologists are agreed that water should not be allowed to enter the ear when a grommet is *in situ*.

In adults
1 **Eustachian catheterization.** (A silver catheter is passed along the floor of the nose, and air is blown into the Eustachian tube. Requires experience and skill.) Simple Politzerization may be effective.
2 **Myringotomy and insertion of drain.** This is carried out as described above. Adenoidectomy will not, as a rule, be required in adults, but examination of the nasopharynx to exclude the presence of tumours is essential and should be carried out under the same anaesthetic. An adult

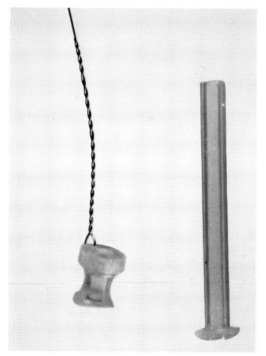

Fig. 47. Tubes inserted through the tympanic membrane for the purpose of ventilating the middle ear. A Teflon tube and a grommet with wire attached.

harbouring a small nasopharyngeal carcinoma may well present with secretory otitis and in other respects be completely symptom-free.

Sequelae

If drainage cannot be effected the fluid is likely to organize, with the formation of fibrous adhesions binding the ossicles one to another, retracting the tympanic membrane and causing conductive deafness (Fig. 48).

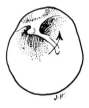

Fig. 48. Retracted tympanic membrane. Note the almost horizontal position of the handle of the malleus.

This condition has been given a number of labels, the most apt of which is perhaps the first:
    Adhesive deafness.
    Chronic middle ear catarrh.
    Eustachian catarrh.
    Chronic adhesive process.
Established adhesive deafness may sometimes be alleviated by tympanotomy, but in the severe and intractable case a hearing-aid may be necessary.

CHAPTER 11
OTOSCLEROSIS

THE early diagnosis of otosclerosis is of importance for the following reasons:

1 Otosclerosis occurs in early adult life when deafness is incapacitating and tragic.
2 Many cases, if treated early, are remediable.
3 Few cases, if treated late, are remediable.

Pathology

Deafness is caused by the formation of new bone in the region of the footplate of the stapes, ankylosing this normally mobile structure. The conduction of vibrations from the tympanic membrane to the cochlea is thus seriously impeded.

Clinical features

1 Usual age of onset 15–30 years.
2 Family history of deafness often present.
3 Formerly females were thought to be affected much more frequently than males but this is now thought to be doubtful.
4 Pregnancy may result in increased deafness.
5 Deafness at first unilateral, later bilateral.
6 Tinnitus often present.
7 Paracusis often present. (Ability to hear conversation more easily in noisy surroundings.)
8 Tympanic membranes normal. (In rapidly progressive cases there may be much hyperaemia of the medial wall of the middle ear, causing a reddish tinge of the tympanic membrane. Schwartze's sign.)
9 Tuning forks—(1) Rinne's test negative (BC > AC). (2) Absolute bone conduction good in early cases, poor in late cases.
10 Audiometry. Air conduction curve is poor. Bone conduction is good. *In late cases the bone conduction deteriorates.*

Treatment

1 Stapedectomy. In a high proportion of cases the hearing may be partially or wholly restored by stapedectomy. After the ossicles have been exposed by reflecting the tympanic membrane forwards, the stapes is removed and replaced by some form of prosthesis. In Schuknecht's operation the prosthesis is formed from stainless steel wire and fat, and in Shea's operation polythene strut and vein-graft. There have been several modifications of these two pioneering methods. Teflon or stainless steel pistons may be used attached at one end to the long process of the incus and inserted through a small hole in the stapes footplate, or alternatively the footplate is sometimes removed completely and the oval window covered with a sheet of Gelfoam which in turn is linked with the incus by means of a steel strut.

The patient is usually kept in hospital for only 3–7 days, and should be warned that the ear is now more vulnerable to very loud noises and sudden pressure changes, which must, as far as possible, be avoided.

2 Fenestration. The fenestration operation was the first great 'break-through' in the surgical treatment of otosclerosis but it is very seldom performed in this present era of stapedectomy. It is, however, referred to at this point as patients who underwent the procedure in its hey-day (1946–56) may consult their medical practitioner for treatment of the cavity. They would at least expect him to have heard of the operation.

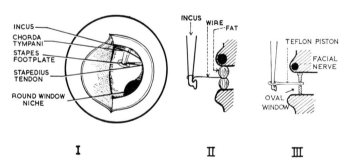

Fig. 49. Stapedectomy. In I is shown the approach to the middle-ear. A semicircular incision has been made in the skin lining the posterior wall of the meatus. A cuff of skin, together with the posterior part of the tympanic membrane, has been reflected forwards. In II the stapes has been replaced by a wire and fat prosthesis after the manner of Schuknecht. In III the crura of the stapes have been removed, a small hole drilled in the footplate, and a Teflon piston inserted.

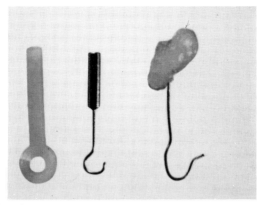

Fig. 50. Three forms of stapes prosthesis used in stapedectomy. Teflon piston, steel piston, fat and wire.

The middle-ear contents are widely exposed by an endaural incision, and after excision of the incus a fenestra is made by diamond burr in the lateral semicircular canal and covered by a mobile membrane derived from the thin meatal skin adjacent to the tympanic membrane (Fig. 51). Sound-waves can now reach the cochlea. Sojourn in hospital 2–3 weeks. The operation cavity may need regular cleansing or the hearing may have deteriorated, in which case there is a possibility that a modified stapedectomy may effect improvement.

3 Hearing-aids and lip-reading. Hearing-aids are usually of enormous benefit in otosclerosis, though most patients prefer to undergo surgical treatment if this is appropriate in their case. In cases where rapid

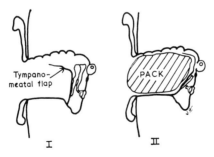

Fig. 51. Fenestration. In I the tympano-meatal flap has been separated. In II the malleus has been decapitated, the incus removed and the lateral semicircular canal fenestrated. A firm pack maintains pressure on the tympano-meatal flap in the post-operative period.

deterioration of hearing seems likely, instruction in lip-reading is of vital importance and should never be neglected.

4   Fluorides. Sodium fluoride has been used in the treatment of certain cases of otosclerosis for a number of years. Owing to its toxicity it should only be administered with extreme care.

CHAPTER 12
EARACHE (OTALGIA)

AURAL CAUSES

Earache is associated with every inflammatory, and many other, conditions of the external ear and middle ear cleft, the most common aural cause of severe earache being **furunculosis, acute otitis media** and **mastoiditis**. **Malignant disease** of the external and middle ear may cause intractable earache.

REFERRED EARACHE

Earache may be referred via the following nerves:
    Auriculo-temporal branch of the trigeminal.

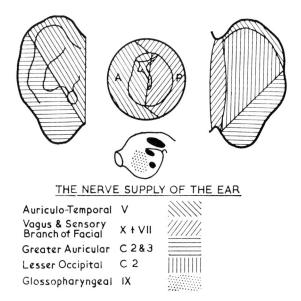

THE NERVE SUPPLY OF THE EAR

Auriculo-Temporal	V	\\\\\
Vagus & Sensory Branch of Facial	X + VII	/////
Greater Auricular	C 2 & 3	≡≡≡
Lesser Occipital	C 2	‖‖‖‖
Glossopharyngeal	IX	∴∴∴

Fig. 52. The nerve supply of the ear.

65

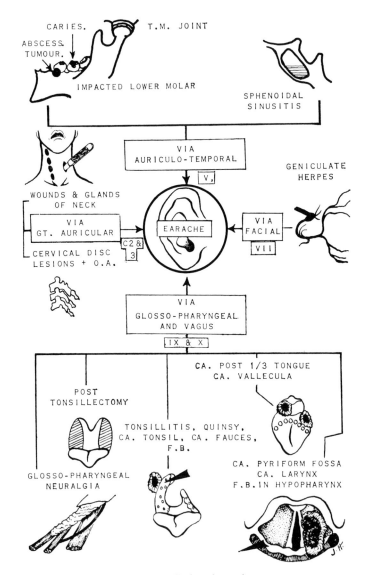

Fig. 53. Referred earache.

Sensory branch of the facial.
Tympanic branch of the glossopharyngeal.
Auricular branch of the vagus.
Lesser occipital, 2nd cervical.
Greater auricular, 2nd + 3rd cervical (Fig. 52).
The causes of referred earache are shown pictorially (Fig. 53), but certain of them deserve special mention on account of their frequency or diagnostic importance.

Post-tonsillectomy earache is very common between the third and sixth days. Armed with this knowledge, do not presume that all post-tonsillectomy earache is referred. *Inspect the ear. Otitis media may be present!*

Impacted lower molars frequently cause prolonged earache, and sometimes trismus. Girls of 18–22 years of age are most commonly afflicted.

Costen's syndrome of aural discomfort, tinnitus and even slight deafness is caused by abnormal stresses in the temporo-mandibular joint. These are usually set up by malocclusion (faulty bite), an abnormality only too often neglected.

Malignant disease of posterior third of tongue, vallecula, fauces, tonsil, lateral pharyngeal wall, larynx and hypopharynx is often associated with earache, which may be an early symptom. *The combination of earache with increasing dysphagia is of sinister portent.*

NOTE: *The problem of* **referred earache** *receives but scant attention in medical training and many doctors are unaware of the frequency of this symptom. Numerous patients drift from one doctor to another receiving ear drops and antibiotics over periods of months or even years, when in fact attention from a dental surgeon for their impacted molars or malocclusion could relieve their problems.*

CHAPTER 13
TINNITUS

TINNITUS, or the complaint of ringing, buzzing, hissing or pulsating noises in the ears or head, is very common and is difficult to relieve.

LOCAL CAUSES

Aural

Tinnitus may be a symptom of *any abnormal condition of the ear*, from a small amount of wax to serious labyrinthine disease. Certain conditions deserve special mention:

Secretory otitis. Tinnitus is an occasional symptom.
Otosclerosis. Surgery often relieves the tinnitus.
Menière's disease. Tinnitus is sometimes almost intolerable.
Glomus tumour. Pulsating tinnitus. Important in diagnosis.
Presbycusis. Tinnitus often accompanies the deafness.

Head and neck

Many of the lesions causing referred otalgia (particularly via the auriculo-temporal or great auricular nerves) also cause tinnitus, e.g.

Impacted lower molars and dental caries.
Temporo-mandibular joint abnormalities (Costen's syndrome).
Wounds of neck and cervical disc lesions.

Arterio-venous aneurysms and some vascular cranial tumours occupy a unique role in causing a clangorous, pulsating and demoralizing din, which can be heard by the examiner, on auscultation, as a bruit.

GENERAL CAUSES

Tinnitus is commonly associated with conditions of general ill-health, systemic abnormality, and toxaemia.

Fevers.

Cardiovascular conditions. (Hypertension, athero-sclerosis.)
Blood diseases. (Anaemias, etc.)
Disease of the C.N.S.
Deficiency diseases.
Drugs. (Quinine, salicylates, ototoxic drugs.)
Alcohol.
Tobacco.

MANAGEMENT

The following concepts may be used to guide the management of tinnitus:
1 Tinnitus due to some simple condition, such as wax in the ear, will be relieved, in most cases, by treating the cause.

2 Many patients (often intelligent) ascribe tinnitus to the presence of a brain tumour, and it is of supreme importance that the doctor, having excluded serious disease, should reassure the patient accordingly.

3 Tinnitus due to chronic disease, or degeneration, e.g. prebycusis, remains with the patient, as a rule, for the test of his life, though if he is of reasonably good 'moral fibre' and is properly handled it should not trouble him unduly. He should be told that the noises will persist, and that if he tries to ignore them they will gradually obtrude less and less on his consciousness. Unfortunately, many doctors, motivated by kindness, tell the sufferer that the noises will disappear, with the result that he listens intently, and finding them still present, concludes that he must have a brain tumour. The anxiety induced by this thought increases his awareness of the tinnitus, and a vicious circle is established.

4 Sedatives and psychotherapy may be necessary in severe cases but nothing could be worse than the giving of sedatives with the implication that they will abolish the tinnitus. 'Just take these pills, and the noises will disappear', is an example of appalling psychology and will result in the patient listening carefully to his tinnitus in an attempt to compare the virtues of one course of pills with another.

An even worse remark not infrequently made to the victims of tinnitus is: 'You've got to learn to live with it'. This in the author's experience, is almost guaranteed to make enemies for life and should never be voiced in connection with any symptoms from chronic headaches to hot flushes.

5. Tinnitus, *per se*, is not an indication for surgical treatment.

CHAPTER 14
VERTIGO

THERE are numerous conditions which may cause vertigo; many of them affect the central nervous system, but in this section we are considering disorders of the vestibular nerve, its ganglion and its end-organ.

> Menière's disease.
> Vestibular neuronitis.
> Benign positional vertigo.
> Vertebro-basilar ischaemia.
> Ototoxic drugs.
> Vascular accidents of the labyrinth.
> Suppurative labyrinthitis.
> Traumatic labyrinthitis.
> Post-operative labyrinthitis.
> Syphilitic labyrinthitis.
> Neoplasm of the labyrinth.
> Acoustic neuroma.
> Geniculate herpes.
> Eustachian obstruction.
> Wax.

MENIÈRE'S DISEASE

Menière's disease is associated with distension of the membranous labyrinth due to increased endolymphatic pressure. The underlying cause is not known though it has now been established that the biochemistry and electrolyte concentrations of the labyrinthine fluids may be abnormal.

The onset usually occurs between 40 and 60 years of age; one ear is affected first, and in about 25 per cent of cases the other ear becomes affected later.

Clinical features are as follows:
1 **Vertigo** is intermittent, the attacks lasting between several minutes

and several hours. They may be preceded by a feeling of pressure in the ear, and are often followed by malaise for several days. The vertigo takes the form of a definite feeling of rotation, not simply unsteadiness.

2　**Nausea** almost always occurs during the attacks.

3　**Vomiting** is frequently present and may be almost uncontrollable.

4　**Deafness** is sensorineural and is usually more marked before and during an attack. In spite of fluctuations it is gradually progressive, and is often associated with intolerable distortion, which to the music-lover may be a worse handicap than the vertigo.

5　**Tinnitus** is a constant trial of the patient's morale, and, like the deafness, may be more marked before and during an attack. It may precede all other symptoms by a period of months or years.

Progress of the disease

The attacks often occur in bouts; for example, there may be a series of three, or four, attacks in a period of a few weeks, followed by freedom from attacks for a period of months or years. With recurring bouts of attacks the affected ear becomes progressively more deaf, and finally the attacks cease.

Then the other ear may commence to misbehave, and the whole gamut is repeated. Often, in the bilateral cases, the second ear commences to be troublesome before the first ear has become completely inert, so attacks are 'fired off' by both labyrinths. A complex situation.

Investigation includes:

1　**Audiometry**
The audiogram shows a sensorineural deafness, the curve often being fairly 'flat', i.e. the losses for high tones and low tones are not greatly dissimilar. Recruitment of loudness is present.

2　**Caloric tests** (Fig. 54). (Fitzgerald and Hallpike technique.)
The patient lies supine with the head flexed forward 30° from the horizontal plane, and is told to look at a small spot on the ceiling directly overhead. Using a douche-can and nozzle, each ear is irrigated with water, first at 30° C., then at 44° C., for 40 seconds. The period of time elapsing between the commencement of irrigation and the cessation of the nystagmus is measured and recorded on a calorigram (Fig. 55). Normally this period is of about 120 seconds' duration. In many cases of Menière's disease the calorigram shows a pattern indicative of canal paresis.

One criticism of caloric testing as described above is that the determination of the actual moment of cessation of the nystagmus is not easy and

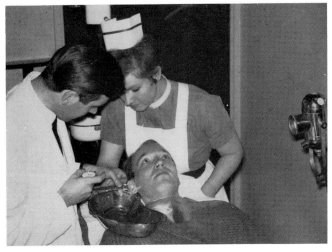

Fig. 54. Caloric tests. See text for description. Note the tangential lighting. Observation of nystagmus using direct illumination from a powerful lamp or head-mirror may be painfully dazzling for the patient.

may vary from one observer to another. This criticism has been answered by the technique of **electronystagmography** in which electrodes attached to the patients frontal and temporal regions pick up action potentials set up in the extrinsic ocular muscles. With suitable amplification a direct recording of the nystagmus may be made.

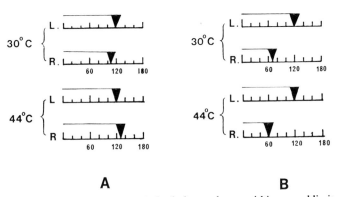

Fig. 55. Two calorigrams (see text). In A the results are within normal limits, but in B there is a well-marked paresis of the right labyrinth which could occur, for example in Menière's disease.

Treatment

Medical

During the attacks, if vomiting is absent, useful preparations are dimenhydrinate (Dramamine) 50 mg four-hourly, chlorpromazine hydrochloride (Largactil) 25 mg six-hourly or prochlorperazine (Stemetil) 5 mg six-hourly. If vomiting is a marked feature of the attack dimenhydrinate 50 mg, or chlorpromazine 25 mg, may be given by intramuscular injection.

Between attacks numerous methods have been advocated, such as:

1 Low fluid and low salt diet.
2 Vasodilators, such as nicotinic acid, 25–100 mg six-hourly, cyclandelate (Cyclospasmol) 200 mg six-hourly or beta-pyridyl carbinol (Ronicol) 25 mg six-hourly.
3 Histamine desensitization.
4 Stellate ganglion block.
5 Phenobarbitone has been used in the treatment of Menière's disease for very many years, and in numerous cases to excellent effect. It is best administered each morning in the form of sustained release capsules (Phenobarbitone Spansule 60 mg or 100 mg). Amylobarbitone 14–45 mg is also of great value.
6 Recently treatment with betahistine hydrochloride (Serc) 8 mg three times daily has been found useful in some cases.

Surgical

1 Labyrinthectomy is very effective in severe unilateral cases. It is contraindicated, as a rule, if the patient has useful hearing in the affected ear, and certainly if the other ear is in any way abnormal.
2 Stellate ganglionectomy.
3 Selective destruction of the labyrinth by the ultrasonic beam. By the use of this method any residual hearing in the treated ear may be preserved.
4 Decompression of the saccus endolymphaticus by the methods of Portman and House, and decompression of the saccule by the method of Fick.

Finally, it must be stressed that the patient with Menière's disease requires continual reassurance from his doctor. The startling suddenness of the attacks, the hideous retching, and, above all, the terrifying insecurity of disorientation in space, together with deafness and cacophonous head noises, contribute to undermine the patient's morale. It is little wonder that many sufferers become severely depressed.

OTHER CAUSES OF LABYRINTHINE VERTIGO

Vestibular neuronitis is occasionally seen in adults, more commonly in the winter months. It is usually regarded as a transient infection (perhaps viral) of the ganglion of Scarpa.

The patient, who may recently have had a febrile illness, has an attack of vertigo similar to the attacks of Menière's disease. The hearing is, however, not affected, though the calorigram pattern is abnormal. Resolution takes place with rest, reassurance and Avomine or Dramamine.

Benign positional vertigo is considered to be due to a degenerative condition of the utricular and saccular maculae, and is seen in adults who may give a history of previous head injury or C.S.O.M. The attacks last a few seconds only and are brought on by head movement—particularly lying back in bed.

The patient is instructed to lie back on a couch and to turn his head to one side. *Any resulting nystagmus is of short duration—a fact which distinguishes the condition from central lesions.* The calorigram pattern is usually within normal limits. Resolution takes place with reassurance and remedial exercises (head turning, etc.).

Vertebro-basilar insufficiency may be the cause of major but momentary attacks of vertigo. In the more severe case there is often marked *atheroma of the vertebral arteries, cervical spondylosis*, or a combination of the two conditions.

The symptom of sudden vertigo may be caused by rotation of the neck or hyper-extension, for example when the patient looks up to admire an architectural feature immediately overhead. On occasions, so instantaneous is the effect of this indiscretion that the patient has a so-called *drop-attack* and falls to the floor.

It should be noted that in vertebro-basilar insufficiency the arterial blood-supply to much of the brain-stem and cerebellum may be impaired and the investigation and treatment of the condition require expert neurological advice.

Ototoxic drugs, such as streptomycin and its analogues, can, in certain cases, destroy labyrinthine function in small doses. The result may be tragic. *Avoid the drugs if possible in any case of impaired renal function.*

Vascular accidents of the labyrinth (e.g. thrombosis, haemorrhage or embolism) cause severe vertigo, passing off after a period of weeks or months.

Suppurative labyrinthitis causes severe vertigo. (See complications of middle ear infection.)

Traumatic labyrinthitis may complicate fractures of the petrous bone, or other labyrinthine injury.

Post-operative labyrinthitis very occasionally follows fenestration.

Syphilitic labyrinthitis. Very rare, but—don't forget the spirochaete.

Neoplasm of the labyrinth. Carcinoma or glomus tumour may spread from the middle ear; there may be direct extension from the cranium or meninges; secondary deposits may occur. The vertigo is severe.

Acoustic neuroma. Vertigo may be slight and transient, or absent. It is not a prominent feature.

Geniculate herpes (herpes oticus, Ramsay Hunt's syndrome), may be associated with transient vertigo.

Eustachian obstruction occasionally causes vertigo.

Wax, when moistened, swells and may compress the tympanic membrane, causing vertigo.

CHAPTER 15
DEAFNESS

CAUSES

THERE is no strict order in the following lists, for the frequency with which the various causes of deafness occur varies considerably from one community to another and from one decade to the next. Nevertheless, some indication of frequency has been given by sub-dividing each list into a 'more common' and a 'less common' group. Even this is a matter of some difficulty; for example—'infection' is one of the more common causes of sensorineural deafness, yet certain infections (syphillis, enteric) are rarely responsible.

Use the lists for reference and with circumspection. Seek first to allot each case of deafness to its respective group—conductive or sensorineural—for with this approach the key to diagnosis, treatment and prognosis is most readily obtained.

CONDUCTIVE	SENSORINEURAL
More Common	**More Common**
Wax.	Presbycusis (senile deafness).
Acute otitis media.	Vascular (haemorrhage, spasm, thrombosis of cochlear vessels).
Chronic otitis media and sequelae.	Infections (measles, mumps, influenza, meningitis, herpes oticus, suppurative labyrinthitis, rarely—syphilis and enteric).
Secretory otitis media and sequelae.	
Meatal infections, f.b., exostoses.	
Barotrauma.	Congenital (maternal rubella and other virus infections, abortifacients, hereditary deafness, haemolytic disease of newborn, anoxia and birth injuries, congenital syphilis).
Otosclerosis.	
Injuries of tympanic membrane.	

CONDUCTIVE	SENSORINEURAL
More Common	**More Common**
	Acoustic trauma (head injuries, sudden blast, e.g. bomb explosion, continued exposure, e.g. small-arms, jet engines, etc.).
	Drugs (streptomycin, neomycin, vancomycin, viomycin, quinine, aspirin).
	Menière's disease.
	Late otosclerosis.
Less Common	**Less Common**
Traumatic ossicular dislocation.	Haemorrhagic (leukaemia, etc.).
Congenital meatal stenosis.	Acoustic nerve tumours.
Nasopharyngeal tumours.	Central nervous system (disseminated sclerosis, secondary deposits, etc.).
Tumours of meatus and middle ear.	Malnutrition (vitamin B deficiency).
	Psychogenic.
	Unknown aetiology.

MANAGEMENT

The management of a number of conditions causing deafness has already been dealt with in other sections, but certain conditions and methods of treatment deserve special mention.

The deaf child

The early diagnosis and treatment of deafness in children of any age is a matter of vital importance, and where a mother suspects deafness in her young child her suspicions are often well founded. The first responsibility of the medical attendant in such cases is to take a detailed history referring to the family, the pregnancy, the labour and the neonatal period. There are numerous simple tests with cup and spoon, whistles, drums and the 'show me' pictures, which are described in the larger text-books and require patience, training and experience but to be brief, the wise practitioner having the slightest suspicion that a young child may be deaf will refer it to an audiology clinic without delay. Here, many hours will be spent by experts not only in testing the child but in giving guidance to parents regarding such matters as hearing-aids and in some cases the necessity for institutional treatment.

Sudden sensorineural deafness

Severe deafness of sudden onset may be unilateral or bilateral. Most of the cases are regarded as being either vascular or viral in origin but in fact numerous different causes have been recorded and in a substantial proportion of cases the cause remains unknown. The forms of treatment employed include vasodilator drugs, cervical sympathetic block and A.C.T.H. or steroids.

It must be borne in mind by the medical student that deafness of this type calls for emergency action, every hour counts, and specialist advice must be sought at once. Sudden bilateral profound hearing loss is a devastating blow, likely to have tragic consequences for the patient and the members of his or her family, and for this reason special organizations exist to give moral support in such cases.

Progressive unilateral deafness

Sensorineural deafness of gradual onset may be the first sign of an acoustic nerve tumour and always merits special investigation including audiometry, caloric tests and radiology in the first place. Later angiography, computerised tomography and brain scan may be required.

Acoustic neuroma is in many cases a curable condition, provided an early diagnosis is made, and for this reason otologists are at pains to exclude it in cases of progressive unilateral deafness.

Hearing-aids

In certain types of sensorineural deafness (cochlear dysfunction) loudness recruitment is a marked feature. This, in simple terms, may be defined as the inability of the patient to tolerate amplification, a common example being the deaf old patient who indignantly asserts 'Don't shout, I'm not deaf'.

The choice of a hearing-aid giving a comfortable yet useful degree of amplification for such patients is often difficult, and a non-electric aid may be preferred. If, however, vanity dictates the use of a small electric aid, an instrument incorporating automatic volume control will probably be necessary. It is fallacious to suppose that a hearing-aid can be 'prescribed' for any patient. Each individual can only be suited by trial with a number of different types of aid, and for this reason it has become customary to refer patients who require small commercial aids to agents who represent not one but a number of manufacturers. *No patient should agree to purchase an aid unless he has been allowed a free trial for a period of at least one week.*

Lip-reading

Instruction in lip-reading plays an important part in the management of deafness, and is a matter of urgency in those who, already moderately deaf, are likely to become severely deaf. It is regrettable that arrangements for lip-reading instruction are all too often neglected.

Cochlear implants

During recent years much research has been undertaken, particularly in the U.S.A. on the implantation of electrodes in the cochlea. By this means the profoundly deaf are in some cases enabled to hear sounds and their powers of communication are thus improved.

However, a great deal of ground has to be covered before cochlear implant surgery becomes commonplace.

CHAPTER 16
FACIAL NERVE PARALYSIS

PARALYSIS of the facial nerve is a subject of fascination to the otologist, and, owing to its frequency and diversity of aetiology, a matter of very considerable importance to workers in all spheres of medical life.

The causes are numerous and may be considered under the following headings.

SUPRANUCLEAR AND NUCLEAR

Cerebral vascular lesions
Poliomyelitis
Cerebral tumours

INFRANUCLEAR

Bell's Palsy
Trauma (Birth injury, fractured temporal bone, surgical).
Tumours (Acoustic neurofibroma, parotid tumours, malignant disease of the middle ear)
Suppuration (Acute or chronic otitis media)
Ramsay Hunt's syndrome
Multiple sclerosis
Guillain-Barré syndrome
Sarcoid

Diagnosis

The patient presents with a varying degree of weakness of the facial muscles and sometimes difficulty in clearing food from the buccogingival sulcus as a result of buccinator paralysis.

Facial asymmetry is accentuated by instructions to close the eyes tightly, to show the teeth or to whistle.

It is important to remember that in **supranuclear lesions** the movements of the *upper part of the face* are likely to be unaffected as the forehead muscles have bilateral cortical representation. Moreover, involuntary movements (e.g. smiling) may be retained even in the *lower face*. A most careful history and aural and neurological examination is essential, including attention to such matters as depressed taste (lesion is above origin of chorda tympani), hyperacusis with loss of the stapedius reflex (lesion is above nerve to stapedius) or reduction of lacrimation (lesion is above geniculate ganglion).

Electrodiagnosis is used in the assessment of the degree of involvement of the nerve and includes *nerve conduction tests* and *electromyography*. A detailed description of the various tests is beyond the scope of this volume, but their application is of very great value as a guide to prognosis and management.

Bell's Palsy (Fig. 56). (Idiopathic facial paralysis)

This, the most common form of facial paralysis, is thought to be due to oedema of the nerve in its vertical course, proximal to the stylomastoid foramen. Aetiology unknown.

It is associated with pain or discomfort in the vicinity of the mastoid and as a rule becomes completely developed within 48 hours of its onset; 90 per cent of all cases make a complete or very satisfactory recovery but some of the remainder are destined to have a truly hideous **deformity**, resulting from the unopposed traction of the contralateral muscles. Other possible sequelae are **crocodile tears** (weeping at meal-times owing to re-routing of parasympathetic fibres from the tympanic plexus to the greater superficial petrosal nerve), **associated movements** (eyelid and mouth movements occur synchronously owing to crossed re-innervation) and **ectropion**.

Treatment is a matter of urgency.

1 A.C.T.H. or oral prednisolone is now advocated by many experts. The course should be commenced within 24 hours. *Do not procrastinate.*

2 **Surgical decompression** of the nerve is advised by some authorities; the decision to operate, and if so—when, is a matter of great difficulty. (And dispute!)

3 **Dental supports** to prevent stretching of the weak facial muscles may be required.

4 **Tarsorrhaphy** may be needed urgently to protect the cornea of the ever open eye.

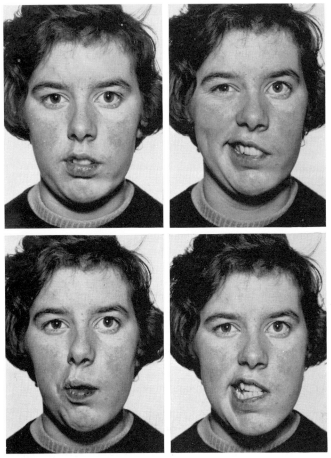

Fig. 56. Left-sided Bell's palsy. In the upper left photograph the face is in repose. Attempts to smile, upper right; to whistle, lower left; and to show the teeth, lower right.

5 Physiotherapy including daily exercise of the facial muscles in front of a mirror help to maintain the patient's morale. Remember, the whole patient needs treatment, not just one half of his face.

6 Plastic surgical techniques including the insertion of fascial slings can do much to improve the appearance in late and severely disfigured cases.

Ramsay Hunt's syndrom. (Herpes oticus: Geniculate herpes, Fig. 57).

A zoster infection of the geniculate ganglion, spreading sometimes to IX and X and very occasionally V, VI or XII.

Severe earache and malaise *precedes* the development of facial palsy with a herpetic eruption of the tympanic membrane, external auditory meatus and concha, and sometimes the palate and pharynx.

Analgesics are essential: Hydroxocobalamin is sometimes used.

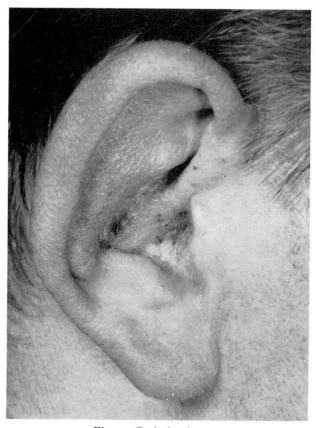

Fig. 57. Geniculate herpes.

Facial palsy in acute or chronic otitis media

A matter for immediate expert advice. Mastoid surgery is usually required.

Traumatic facial palsy

This may result from fractures of the temporal bone or occur as a result of surgery. Otological advice should be sought early in cases of head injury associated with deafness, bleeding from the ear or facial palsy as decompression of the nerve or grafting from the lateral cutaneous nerve of thigh may be required. In some cases faciohypoglossal anastomosis has been carried out.

CHAPTER 17
CLINICAL EXAMINATION OF THE NOSE
AND NASOPHARYNX

Head-mirror. Skill in the use of the head-mirror is acquired more readily if the following details receive attention:

1 The mirror should have a focal length of 8–12 inches and a central hole of not less than $\frac{1}{2}$ inch diameter (Fig. 58).

2 Assuming the examiner prefers to use his right eye, the source of light should be placed about 6 inches away from and behind the patient's left ear. **The beam of light must be directed at the mirror** (Fig. 59).

3 In order to focus the mirror the examiner should then **close his left eye,** look through the hole with his right eye at the tip of the patient's nose, and without moving his head adjust the mirror so that the spot of light falls on the same area. The left eye may then be opened. When some experience has been acquired, the practice of closing one eye for focusing may be abandoned, but it is invaluable to the beginner.

Anterior rhinoscopy is accomplished with Thudichum's speculum (Fig. 60), and whichever method of holding this instrument is adopted the following details should be kept in mind:

1 The hand should be steadied on the patient's forehead.

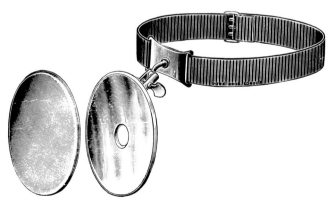

Fig. 58. Head-mirror.

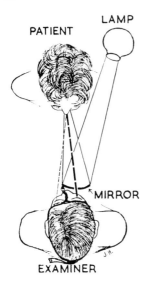

Fig. 59. Head-mirror in use. The examiner can see far into any cavity with his right eye, with which he is looking *through* the hole in the mirror. He is also looking past the mirror with his left eye.

2   The septum is extremely sensitive, so the blade on this side must be carefully controlled.

3   The examiner's line of vision must remain unobstructed by his fingers.

The anterior parts of the septum and middle and inferior turbinates are usually visible. The inferior turbinate is often mistaken for a polyp by the inexperienced, who, if in doubt, may confirm its rigid structure by gentle palpation with a probe.

Posterior rhinoscopy is carried out with a post-nasal mirror of about 12 mm diameter (Fig. 61).

1   The face of the mirror is gently warmed and the back tested on the hand.

2   A Lack's tongue depressor held in the left hand is introduced.

3   The light is focused on the posterior pharyngeal wall and the patient is instructed to keep his mouth open, but to attempt to breathe through the nose. (The soft palate immediately moves forward, away from the posterior pharyngeal wall.)

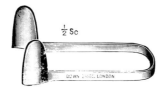

Fig. 60.
Thudichum's speculum.

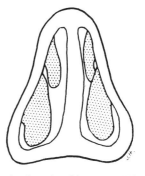

Fig. 62. Anterior rhinoscopy. (The septum is slightly deflected to the left.)

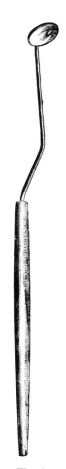

Fig. 61.
Post-nasal mirror.

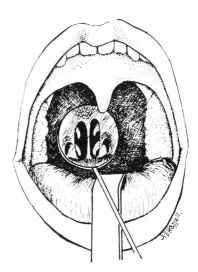

Fig. 63. Posterior rhinoscopy.

4   The mirror is introduced behind and to one side of the uvula, care being taken to avoid contact with the uvula, tongue, fauces or pharyngeal wall.

Posterior rhinoscopy is not easy, and in some individuals unrewarding. Children of 6–12 are often surprisingly good subjects, but seeing the mirror being warmed may inspire them with fear, so this should be done surreptitiously by a third person.

Normal structures visible under good conditions are: the openings of the Eustachian tubes, the posterior extremity of the septum, and, on either side, the choanal openings with the posterior ends of the inferior and middle turbinates therein, the roof of the nasopharynx, and, if present, adenoids (Fig. 63).

Fibre-optic instruments are available for examination of the nasal cavities and in some cases their use enables the examination of areas which could not be reached by the older methods. They are of considerable use in medical photography.

CHAPTER 18
FOREIGN BODY IN THE NOSE

CHILDREN between the ages of 1–4 years sometimes insert foreign bodies into one or both nostrils. The objects of their choice may be hard, such as buttons, beads or ball-bearings, or soft, such as paper, cotton wool, rubber or other vegetable materials, and the latter being as a rule more irritating, tend to give rise to symptoms more quickly.

The child, however intelligent, is unlikely to indicate that a foreign body is present in his nose; he may, in fact, deny the possibility, in order to avoid rebuke.

Clinical picture

1 A fretful child.
2 Unilateral evil-smelling nasal discharge, sometimes blood-stained.
3 Excoriation around the nostril.
4 Occasionally, X-ray evidence.

Dangers

1 Injury from clumsy attempts at removal by unskilled persons.
2 Local spread of infection→sinusitis or meningitis.
3 Inhalation of foreign body→lung abscess.

Management—casualty officers in particular should be alive to the possibility of nasal foreign bodies in small children. The child's mother may say that she suspects a foreign body, and, in fact, the presence of a foreign body may be obvious. On the other hand, there is often an element of uncertainty, and full reassurance cannot be given until every step has been taken to reveal the true state of affairs. *When in doubt, call in expert advice.*

In the case of a co-operative child it may be possible, with head-mirror (or lamp) and Thudichum's speculum to see, and with small nasal forceps or blunt hooks to remove, the foreign body without general anaesthetic. Local analgesia and decongestion are helpful and may be applied in the form of a small cotton-wool swab wrung out in cocaine 10 per cent mixed with an equal quantity of 1/1000 adrenaline. Extreme care is necessary.

A refractory child should, from the onset, be regarded as a case necessitating general anaesthesia. This must be administered by an experienced anaesthetist, and it is usual to employ an endotracheal tube. The surgeon may then remove the foreign body and need have no fear that it will enter the trachea.

Rarely, an adult complaining of nasal obstruction is found to have a large concretion blocking one side of the nose. This is a **rhinolith,** and consists of many layers of calcium and magnesium salts, which have formed around a small central nucleus. The latter often contains a foreign body.

CHAPTER 19
INJURIES OF THE NOSE

THE nose may be injured in various forms of sport, in personal assaults, and in traffic accidents.

Injury of the nose may result in one or a combination of several of the following:

1 Epistaxis (dealt with later).
2 Fractures of the nasal bones.
3 Fracture or dislocation of the septum.
4 Septal haematoma.

FRACTURE OF THE NASAL BONES

The fracture is often simple but comminuted. It may be compound with an open wound in the skin over the nasal bones.

Symptoms and signs

1 Swelling and discoloration of the skin and subcutaneous tissues covering the nasal bones and in the vicinity.
2 Tenderness.
3 Mobility of the nose.
4 Deformity. *This may or may not be present and is of importance in deciding upon treatment.*

Treatment

First, treat epistaxis.

An open wound should be cleansed and, if necessary, sutured. X-rays should be taken, as these may be of medico-legal value. Then look for deformity, the presence or absence of which is now your guide. If deformity is absent no manipulative treatment or splintage is required. If deformity is present, i.e. the nose is squashed against the face or points to left or right, reduction of the fracture will be necessary. *There is an optimum time for this manipulation to be carried out.*

When to reduce the fracture. There have been instances when stalwart types on the football field have sustained fractures of the nose which have there and then been reduced manually by a medical attendant. As a rule, however, the patient presents himself a few hours after the injury, by which time oedema of the soft tissues precludes satisfactory manipulation. In this case no attempt should be made to manipulate the nose until 3–5 days after the injury. This is the optimum time. After this the bony fragments commence to unite with speed, and by the time a further 5–6 days have passed it may be exceedingly difficult to reduce the fracture and restore the nose to its former shapely appearance.

Reduction of fractured nasal bones at the optimum time

The nasal mucosa is thoroughly sprayed with a cocaine and adrenaline mixture (10 per cent Cocaine, 1/1000 Adrenalin, equal parts).

The patient is given a general anaesthetic, with endotracheal tube; anything short of this, such as a 'whiff of gas' or 'shot in the arm' is dangerous, for blood may very easily be inhaled.

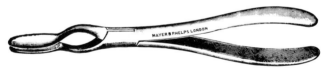

Fig. 64. Walsham's forceps.

The manipulation is carried out with elevators and Walsham's forceps (Fig. 64), one blade of which may be inserted in the nose whilst the other blade lies on the skin. The depressed nasal bone may thus be elevated into position. No splintage is necessary, though a light carapace of plaster bandage is sometimes applied for protection during recovery from anaesthesia.

The late case of fractured nasal bones, in which the patient presents himself months or even years after the injury, is a different problem. The skin and soft tissues must be elevated from the bony skeleton via incisions inside the nares, and the bones then re-fractured, before their former alignment can be restored. The various surgical techniques involved are grouped under the term 'Rhinoplasty' of which a clear account with good bibliography is given by Bull and Walter in *Recent Advances in Otolaryngolo*— (see Chapter 48, 'Further Reading and Higher Qualifications'.)

FRACTURE OR DISLOCATION OF THE SEPTUM

In this case the blow has resulted in a severe deviation of the septum, causing a varying degree of nasal obstruction.

The treatment is by submucous resection of the septum or septoplasty after a period of several weeks.

SEPTAL HAEMATOMA

Sometimes, soon after a punch on the nose, the victim complains of very severe or complete nasal obstruction. This may be caused by a septal haematoma—the result of haemorrhage between the two sheets of muco-perichondrium covering the septum. It is often (but not always) associated with a fracture of the septum.

The appearance is quite distinctive. Both nasal passages are obliterated by a boggy, pink or dull red swelling replacing the septum.

Treatment—may be expectant in the case of a very small haematoma, but a large one requires incision (in Little's area), evacuation of the clot, the insertion of a drain, and nasal packing to approximate the septal coverings of muco-perichondrium. Antibiotic cover should be given in an attempt to avert the development of a septal abscess. The patient should be warned that deformity of the nose may ultimately occur. (The outcome of necrosis of the cartilage.)

CHAPTER 20

EPISTAXIS

EPISTAXIS (nasal haemorrhage) is a common condition. It may be extremely serious, and it behoves every house surgeon, casualty officer or general practitioner to have clear-cut ideas regarding its causation and the steps which should be taken to arrest it.

ANATOMY

Bleeding usually arises from the nasal septum, which is supplied by the following vessels:

> Anterior ethmoidal artery.
> Posterior ethmoidal artery.
> Greater palatine artery (terminal branch).
> Sphenopalatine artery (septal branch).
> Superior labial artery (septal branch).

These vessels anastomose on the anterior part of the septum in Little's area—frequently the site of epistaxis (Fig. 65).

Epistaxis is less common from the lateral wall of the nose, which is supplied largely by the main trunk of the sphenopalatine artery, and the ethmoidal arteries.

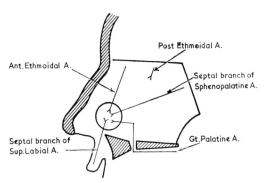

Fig. 65. The blood supply of the nasal septum. Little's area is within the circle.

AETIOLOGY

The causes of epistaxis are numerous. For the purpose of classification they may be divided into two groups—local and general.

LOCAL	GENERAL
'Spontaneous'.	**Cardiovascular conditions:**
Trauma.	Hypertension.
Post-operative.	High venous tension (mitral
Tumours of nose and	stenosis).
sinuses.	**Abnormal conditions of blood**
Hereditary telangiectasia.	**or vessels:**
Atrophic rhinitis.	Leukaemia.
	Anaemia.
	Purpura.
	Haemophilia.
	Scurvy.
	Hodgkin's disease.
	Vitamin K deficiency.
	Fevers:
	Enteric.
	Influenza.
	Smallpox.

What are the common types of epistaxis which the practitioner is likely to meet in everyday life? They are two in number—one from the 'local' group and one from the 'general' group.

'Spontaneous' epistaxis:

Common in children, adolescents, young adults (usually female).
Arises from Little's area.
Probably often associated with slight trauma or infection.
Usually easy to stop.
Tends to recur.

Hypertensive epistaxis:

A later age group.
Arises far back in the nose.

Often extremely difficult to stop.

May recur.

TREATMENT

A. **Pressure and posture.** The patient, in a sitting position with the head flexed slightly forwards, presses with his finger against the bleeding side of the nose for 10 minutes. The mouth is kept open, swallowing is forbidden, and the patient dribbles into a bowl under the chin. This is a modification of Trotter's method.

B. **Anterior nasal packing**—is the next step if (A) above is not successful.

The side which is bleeding is sprayed with a cocaine and adrenaline mixture (10 per cent cocaine, 1/1000 adrenaline, equal parts).

The nose is now packed with $\frac{1}{2}$-inch ribbon-gauze moistened with the same solution.

With Tilley's forceps (Fig. 66) the ribbon is first passed along the floor of the nose to the back in a loop, and then built up in successive loops from the floor upwards (Fig. 67). By this means even pressure is exerted on the

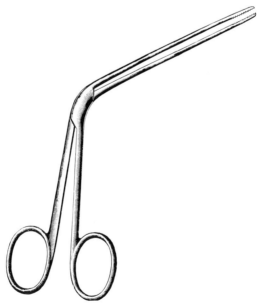

Fig. 66. Tilley's nasal dressing forceps.

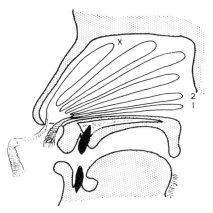

Fig. 67. Insertion of anterior nasal pack. 1 is the first loop, 2—the second, and X—the last.

whole nasal mucosa, and the posterior parts of the pack are not likely to be swallowed. The pack may be left for 24 hours, or longer if the patient is under hospital supervision and antibiotic cover. An inflatable rubber bag is sometimes used in lieu of a gauze pack.

C. **Post-nasal plugging**—may be necessary if the bleeding is arising very far back and cannot be controlled by an anterior nasal pack.

The plug consists of a tightly compressed ball of gauze about the size of a walnut, firmly secured by stitches to the centre of a piece of tape about 2 feet in length (Fig. 68). The directions for its insertion are as follows:

1 Spray the nose with cocaine and adrenaline mixture.

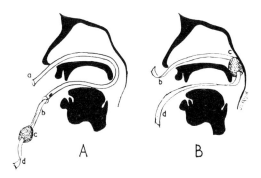

Fig. 68. Insertion of post-nasal plug. A. First stage. B. Second stage. *a*. Catheter. *b*. 'Leading' tape. *c*. Plug. *d*. Trailing tape.

2   Pass along the floor of the nose on the more profusely bleeding side, a soft rubber catheter.

3   Look in the mouth, seize the catheter as it passes into the pharynx, and draw the tip of the catheter out through the mouth. Avoid injury to the uvula.

4   Attach one end of the tape to the tip of the catheter and draw this back through the nose.

5   When the plug reaches the back of the mouth, push it behind the soft palate with the tip of your finger. Avoid being bitten.

6   Exert moderate tension on the 'leading' end of the tape by drawing it round the side of the face and attaching it firmly thereto with adhesive tape. The 'trailing' end of the tape should be led out of the corner of the mouth and attached without tension.

7   If necessary, a firm anterior nasal pack may now be inserted without any danger of its being swallowed.

A patient acting as host to a post-nasal plug should be in hospital and on antibiotics. The plug may be left for 24 hours, and may then be removed by cutting the leading tape and gently hauling on the trailing tape.

In spite of the fact that packing and plugging has been used as the classical method of arresting epistaxis there has, during recent years, been a definite trend towards treatment by sedation only. The patient is nursed in bed in a well propped-up position and it must be emphasized that careful observation, usually under hospital conditions, is essential. The great advantage of this method, which is often successful, is that trauma of the delicate nasal mucous membrane caused by packing—for example with ribbon gauze—is avoided.

D. **Surgical methods** of controlling epistaxis, rarely resorted to, are as follows:

Submucous resection of the septum (when the bleeding vessel is behind a spur or deviation).

Ligation of the ethmoidal arteries (via the orbital periosteum).

Ligation of the maxillary artery (via the maxillary antrum).

RECURRENT SPONTANEOUS EPISTAXIS FROM LITTLE'S AREA

A common problem in the surgery or out-patient department. The patient has recurrent bouts of epistaxis, which are fairly readily controlled. She presents 'between' bleeds seeking relief from her embarrassing tendency.

Cocainize Little's area by first spraying with the usual cocaine and adrenaline mixture, and by leaving in contact with the area for 10 minutes a pledget of cotton wool soaked in the same solution.

Having removed the wool swab, cauterize the vessel by touching the area lightly with one of the following:

1   A very small cotton-wool swab soaked in trichloracetic acid (saturated solution) and mounted firmly on a Jobson Horne cotton-wool carrier. Be very careful with this acid. Do not slop it about, or allow it to go anywhere other than on the intended site.

2   A bead of fused chromic acid on a wire probe.

3   The galvano-cautery at dull red heat. (Many patients find this method frightening.)

NOTE: *Epistaxis may well be a manifestation of widespread disease, it may be exceedingly serious calling for expert treatment and numerous blood transfusions. It may kill.*

CHAPTER 21
THE NASAL SEPTUM

SEPTAL DEFLECTION

DEFLECTED or deviated nasal septum (D.N.S.) is a common cause of nasal obstruction, and in most cases may be corrected by surgery, with excellent results.

AETIOLOGY

Most cases of D.N.S. result from trauma, either recent, or long forgotten, or perhaps even in the birth canal. Buckling of the septum becomes more pronounced as time passes, and this explains why a fall on the nose in childhood may not cause symptoms for 20 or more years.

CLINICAL FEATURES

Symptoms

1 Nasal obstruction. May be unilateral or bilateral.
2 Recurrent sinus infection. This may be due to pressure of septal convexity on the middle turbinate, resulting in obstruction of the sinus ostia. Alternatively, the middle turbinate on the *concave* side of the septum may undergo hypertrophy and interfere with sinus drainage.
3 Headache. Due to mal-ventilation of the frontal sinus. The so-called 'vacuum' headache.

Signs

1 Septal deformity is immediately seen on examination with a nasal speculum. There may be an S-shape deflection obstructing both passages; angular deviations and sharp spurs result from trauma (Fig. 69).
2 There may be signs of sinus infection.

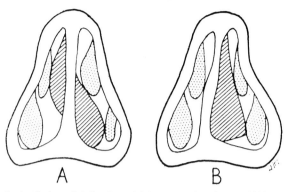

Fig. 69. A. An S-shaped deflection with hypertrophy of one middle turbinate and the contralateral inferior turbinate.
B. A severe traumatic deflection.

TREATMENT

If symptoms are minimal and only a minor degree of deviation is present, relief may be obtained by the regular use of a simple nasal douche.

Cases of moderate or severe deviation must be corrected surgically by submucous resection or septoplasty. A brief account of submucous resection is given first as it has been performed for many years and is still widely practised. However, many surgeons rightly consider that in the majority of septal deviations septoplasty is more appropriate.

Submucous resection (S.M.R.) is a common nasal operation in adults, but should, if possible, be avoided in children, as it may result in depression of the nasal ridge.

The nasal cavities are first packed with cocaine and adrenaline solution for 40 minutes. Under general anaesthesia an incision is made on one side of the septum in the muco-perichondrium, which is then elevated from the underlying bone and cartilage. The incision is deepened and the muco-perichondrium on the other side elevated (Fig. 70).

Deflected cartilage and bone may now be removed by punch forceps, after which the two sheets of muco-perichondrium are allowed to fall together in the mid-line. Pressure on the flaps is maintained by packs or splints, which are removed after 24 hours. Sojourn in hospital 7–9 days.

Complications, which are rare, can be effectively treated; they include septal haematoma, septal perforation, epistaxis and depression of the nasal ridge or tip.

Septoplasty or septal reposition as an alternative to the classical

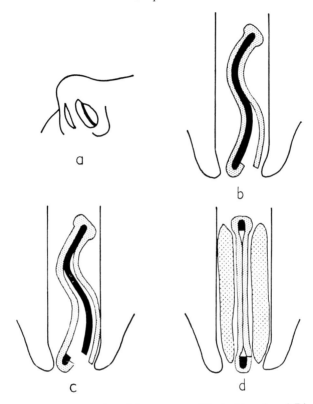

Fig. 70. Submucous resection of the septum. *a*. The incision. *b*, *c*, *d*. Diagrammatic transverse sections showing the separation of muco-perichondrium (stippled) from underlying cartilage and bone (black). In *d*, the packs (cross-hatched) have been inserted.

S.M.R. has gained ground during recent years. As the name implies the major portion of the cartilaginous septum is *repositioned* rather than removed, thereby avoiding the embarrassing deformity of tip or ridge depression which occasionally follows resection.

SEPTAL PERFORATION

AETIOLOGY

Perforation of the nasal septum is most common in its anterior cartilaginous part and may result from the following conditions:

Post-operative (particularly S.M.R.).

Trauma (gunshot wounds, tribal customs, etc.).
Nose-picking (ulceration occurs first, perforation later).
Inhalation of fumes of chrome salts.
Cocaine addiction (sniffing 'snow').
Rodent ulcer.
Lupus.
Malignant granuloma.
Syphilis (the gumma affects the entire septum and nasal bones with
   resulting deformity).

CLINICAL FEATURES

Symptoms consist of epistaxis and crusting, which may cause considerable obstruction. Occasionally whistling on inspiration or expiration is present. Frequently the subject is symptom-free.

Signs. A perforation is readily seen and often has unhealthy edges, covered with large crusts.

TREATMENT

If there is any doubt regarding the pathology a biopsy is taken.

It is sometimes helpful to remove the cartilaginous edges of the perforation, leaving mucous membrane, which can then fall in and cover remaining cartilage adequately.

CHAPTER 22
SOME NASAL INFECTIONS
(EXCLUDING SINUSITIS)

ACUTE CORYZA

THE common cold is probably of virus origin, with secondary bacterial infection.

Local nasal treatment (drops, sprays, etc.) should be avoided in the early stages, in order to minimize the risk of otitis media. Later, medicated steam inhalations are of value.

The prolonged use of nasal decongestants should be vigorously discouraged, owing to their adverse effect on the nasal mucosa (vasomotor rhinitis medicamentosa).

VESTIBULITIS

Infection of the skin of the nasal vestibule is sometimes found in nose-picking children or debilitated adults. Foreign body, sinusitis and systemic disease, e.g. anaemia should be excluded.

Ung. hydrarg. nitratis. dil. as a local application is invaluable.

FURUNCULOSIS

Boils sometimes occur following interference with the nasal vibrissae. The tip of the nose becomes tense, red and tender. *Incision or squeezing must be avoided; cavernous sinus thrombosis has followed such interference.* Antibiotic treatment is advisable, and in recurrent cases the urine should be tested for sugar, and staphyloccal vaccines tried.

NASAL DIPHTHERIA

This is rare but should be suspected in a child having a blood-stained nasal discharge with excoriation of the skin around the vestibule. The nose contains crusts and membrane. Foreign body must be excluded. Toxaemia is usually mild, but the condition is highly infectious, and vigorous treatment with antitoxin and penicillin must be instituted.

ATROPHIC RHINITIS (OZAENA)

Though now uncommon in communities enjoying the affluence of Western civilization, atrophic rhinitis is still seen occasionally. The nasal mucosa undergoes atrophy, and the nose becomes filled with crusts which emit a nauseating stench and may render the patient a social outcast. Epistaxis and headache occur, but the patients, usually women, are seldom conscious of the foul effluvium which surrounds them.

Little is known regarding the aetiology, though hormonal dysfunction probably plays a part.

The nose should be douched or syringed with an alkaline solution daily, and thereafter sprayed with an oily solution of Oestradiol. By this means the smell may be controlled, though the disease is rarely cured.

CHAPTER 23
MAXILLARY SINUSITIS

SOME ANATOMY AND PHYSIOLOGY

THE maxillary sinus is pyramidal in shape, and in the adult has a capacity of 15 ml (approx.).

Its ostium, in the upper part of its medial wall, opens into the hiatus semilunaris of the middle meatus (Fig. 71).

The maxillary sinus (antrum) is related:

Superiorly to the infra-orbital vessels and nerve and orbital contents.

Inferiorly to the lateral part of the hard palate, and the roots of the second pre-molar and first two molar teeth.

Posteriorly to the pterygopalatine fossa containing the maxillary artery.

Medially to the lateral nasal wall in its middle and inferior meatus and the naso-lachrymal duct.

Anteriorly to the bucco-alveolar sulcus.

The antrum is lined with ciliated columnar epithelium containing numerous mucous cells. Mucus is swept by the cilia in a continual blanket towards the ostium and thence into the nose.

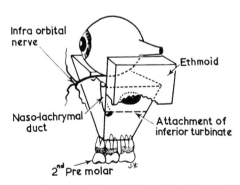

Fig. 71. Diagram showing some of the relations of the right maxillary sinus. Part of the middle turbinate has been removed to show the sinus ostium.

ACUTE INFECTION

AETIOLOGY

Most cases of acute maxillary sinusitis are secondary to the nasal infection of:

1 Influenza.
2 Common cold.
3 Measles, whooping-cough, etc.

In about 10 per cent of cases the infection arises from the pre-molar or molar teeth, as in:

1 Apical abscess.
2 Dental extraction.

Occasionally infection follows the entry of infected material as a result of trauma, as in:

1 Gunshot wounds.
2 Fractures.
3 Diving. (Water is forced through ostium.)

Predisposing factors to infection are:

1 Poor drainage, e.g. septal deviations.
2 Virulent infection.
3 Low resistance of patient.

PATHOLOGY

The organisms concerned are usually streptococci or staphylococci, but in dental infections anaerobic organisms are often present.

The mucous membrane lining the antrum becomes inflamed and oedematous, and pus forms. If the ostium if obstructed by oedematous mucosa the antrum becomes filled with pus under pressure—'empyema of the antrum'.

CLINICAL FEATURES

Symptoms

1 Patient usually has an upper respiratory infection or gives a history of dental infection or extraction.

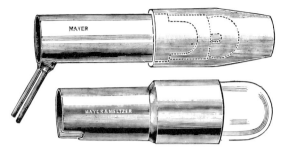

Fig. 72. Sinus transilluminator.

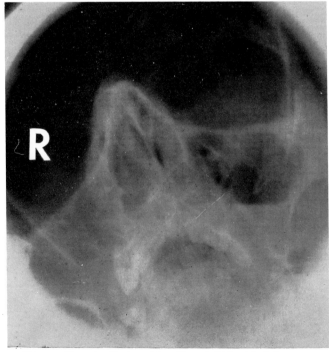

Fig. 73. X-ray in tilted position. Note fluid level in left antrum.

2 Pain in the face. Sometimes referred supraorbitally. The pain is often throbbing and may be made worse by head movements, walking or stooping.

3 Nasal obstruction.

4 Nasal discharge may be very scanty if ostium is blocked. The complaint of a bad smell suggests 'dental' infection of the sinus.

Signs

1 Pyrexia is often present.

2 Tenderness may be elicited over the antrum.

3 Mucopurulent discharge may be seen as a yellow streak under the middle turbinate or in the nasopharynx.

4 Maxillary antrum fails to transilluminate clearly.

5 X-rays show opacity and sometimes a fluid level (Fig. 73).

6 An oro-antral fistula may be present in cases of dental origin.

THREE IMPORTANT RULES

1 SWELLING OF THE CHEEK IS VERY RARE IN MAXILLARY SINUSITIS.

2 SWELLING OF THE CHEEK IS MOST COMMONLY OF DENTAL ORIGIN.

3 SWELLING OF THE CHEEK AS A RESULT OF ANTRAL DISEASE USUALLY IMPLIES CARCINOMA OF THE MAXILLARY ANTRUM.

TREATMENT

1 Bed is advisable.

2 Penicillin should be given in severe cases.

3 Nasal decongestion must be achieved as soon as possible by the use of 2 per cent ephedrine or 1/1000 privine nasal drops, followed by menthol inhalations 4-hourly.

4 Analagesics.

In most cases resolution takes place, but occasionally discomfort persists in spite of conservative treatment, and antrum puncture and washout may be necessary. It should be avoided if possible in acute maxillary sinusitis, and should not be carried out in the early stages.

COMPLICATIONS

1 Spread to other sinuses, e.g. frontal sinus.

2 Otitis media.
3 Downward spread laryngitis or pneumonia.
4 Chronicity.

CHRONIC INFECTION

AETIOLOGY

Most cases of acute maxillary sinusitis resolve completely, but in some the infection becomes chronic. Factors predisposing to chronicity are as follows:

1 Poor drainage, e.g. septal deviations.
2 Virulent infection.
3 Low resistance of patient.
4 'Dental' infections often chronic.
5 Inadequate treatment of acute infection.

PATHOLOGY

1 Flora becomes mixed.
2 Mucous membrane lining the antrum becomes hypertrophic and sometimes polypoidal.
3 Nasal mucous membrane hypertrophic.

CLINICAL FEATURES

Symptoms

1 Nasal obstruction. (On the affected side.)
2 Nasal and post-nasal discharge ('post-nasal drip').
3 Huskiness is often present (rhinitic laryngitis).
4 Cachosmia in infections of dental origin.

Signs

1 Mucopurulent discharge under the middle turbinate or in the naso-pharynx.
2 Antrum fails to transilluminate clearly.
3 X-rays show opacity or fluid level or thickened lining mucosa.
4 An oro-antral fistula may be present in cases of dental origin.

TREATMENT

A. **Antrum puncture and lavage.** (Proof puncture: Antrum wash-out, etc.)

1   The nasal muscosa is sprayed with a mixture of equal parts of 10 per cent cocaine and 1/1000 adrenaline. A small pledget of wool moistened with the same solution and mounted on a silver wire probe is then inserted under the inferior turbinate and left for 15 minutes.

2   A Lichtwitz trocar and cannula (Fig. 74) is now inserted under the inferior turbinate with its tip as high as possible, and about 1 to $1\frac{1}{2}$ inches from the nasal orifice.

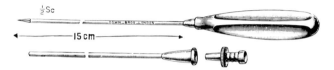

Fig. 74. Lichtwitz trocar and cannula.

3   The handpiece of the trocar is now swung across the midline to the opposite side, and with a slightly rotatory motion the instrument is pushed through the antro-nasal wall, 'aiming' in the direction of the outer canthus (Fig. 75). The trocar is removed.

4   The patient is now instructed to bend forwards, open his mouth and breathe only through the latter. The antrum is irrigated with sterile normal saline by means of a Higginson's syringe, effluent being collected

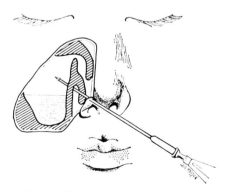

Fig. 75. Diagram to show position of trocar and cannula in proof puncture of the right antrum.

in a receiver. Specimens should be sent for bacteriological investigation.

NOTE: *Swelling of the cheek or orbit may occur if the cannula is incorrectly placed. Fatal air-embolism may follow the forcible injection of air.*

Antrum puncture and lavage should be repeated after a period of four or five days and again if necessary. In many cases the infection resolves and the effluent becomes clear by the third or fourth wash-out.

If an organism can be isolated and its sensitivity determined, lavage followed by the instillation of the appropriate antibiotic is often of value.

If infection is still present after six wash-outs, it is advisable to proceed to the next 'stage'—intra-nasal antrostomy.

B. Intra-nasal antrostomy

Under general anaesthesia an opening is made in the antro-nasal wall (under the inferior turbinate) and enlarged by punch forceps (Fig. 76).

From the fourth day, lavage is carried out daily with a Rose's cannula. This treatment causes minimal discomfort and may be continued by the patient himself after leaving hospital. Sojourn in hospital 5–6 days.

If resolution fails to take place, it is advisable to proceed to the next 'stage'—the Caldwell-Luc operation.

C. The Caldwell-Luc operation (Radical antrostomy)

This has three distinct advantages:

1   The interior of the maxillary antrum can be thoroughly inspected and all diseased tissue, polypi, etc., removed.
2   A very large opening or antrostome can be made in the antro-nasal wall, with minimal trauma to the nasal mucosa. (This may not always be attainable in the intra-nasal operation.)

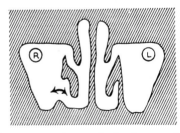

Fig. 76. Intra-nasal antrostomy. An opening has been made in the antro-nasal, or lateral, nasal wall on the right side.

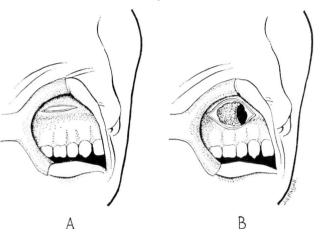

A   B

Fig. 77. Caldwell-Luc. A. An incision has been made in the mucoperiosteum of the right canine fossa. B. A large window has been made in the anterior antral wall. An opening has also been made in the medial wall of the antrum providing free drainage into the nose.

3   Free acccess to the ethmoidal cells is obtained, and, if necessary, they may be opened.

Under general anaesthesia an incision is made in the mucoperiosteum of the canine fossa. A window into the antrum is made in the underlying bone, and diseased tissue removed (Fig. 77).

The antro-nasal wall under the attachment of the inferior turbinate is now removed, with the formation of a large antrostome into the nose. The canine fossa wound does not require sutures and heals rapidly. Sojourn in hospital 8–10 days.

CHAPTER 24
FRONTAL SINUSITIS

ACUTE INFECTION

AETIOLOGY

Infection of the frontal sinus usually occurs as a complication of common cold or influenza, and is often associated with ethmoidal and maxillary sinus infection.

It is predisposed to by any abnormality interfering with the drainage of the frontal sinus, e.g. septal deviation or large middle turbinate.

CLINICAL FEATURES

The symptoms and signs are similar to those of acute maxillary sinusitis, with the following additional features:

1 The pain is mainly supra-orbital.
2 The pain may be periodic. (Present in the morning. Very severe at mid-day. Subsides during the afternoon.)
3 Acute tenderness is elicited by upward pressure under the floor of the sinus or by percussion of its anterior wall.
4 Oedema of the upper eyelid may be present.
5 X-rays show opacity or fluid level in frontal sinus, and usually opacity of ethmoids and maxillary sinus.

TREATMENT

1 Bed.
2 Penicillin should be given early.
3 Nasal decongestion. (See maxillary sinusitis, acute.)
4 Analgesics. (Full dosage necessary.)
5 In fulminating cases, with increasing oedema of the eyelid, the frontal sinus must be drained. Under general anaesthesia an incision is made below the medial $\frac{1}{3}$ of the eyebrow and a small trephine opening made into the sinus. A drainage tube is inserted.

COMPLICATIONS (Fig. 78)

1 **Orbital complications** (cellulitis or abscess) are characterized by diplopia, marked oedema of the eyelids, chemosis of the conjunctiva, and sometimes proptosis. Resolution usually follows intensive antibiotic therapy and local drainage.

2 **Meningitis,** extradural and subdural abscesses may occur and should be treated as neuro-surgical emergencies.

3 **Cerebral abscess** (frontal lobe) deserves special mention in view of the insidious nature of its development. Any patient who has a history of recent frontal sinus infection and complains of headaches, is apathetic, or exhibits any abnormality of behaviour, should be suspected of harbouring a frontal lobe abscess.

4 **Osteomyelitis of the frontal bone** is characterized by persistent headache and oedema of the scalp in the vicinity of the frontal sinus. X-ray signs are late, and by the time they become apparent osteomyelitis is well established. Sequestration may occur, and intensive antibiotic therapy combined with removal of diseased bone is necessary.

5 **Cavernous sinus thrombosis** is very rare. Proptosis, chemosis and ophthalmoplegia characterize this sinister complication.

RECURRENT AND CHRONIC INFECTION

Some individuals suffer from recurrent attacks of acute frontal sinusitis, and in time the mucous membrane lining the sinus and the fronto-nasal

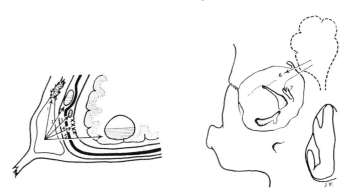

Fig. 78. Complications of frontal sinusitis. 1. Osteomyelitis. 2. Extradural abscess. 3. Subdural abscess. 4. Meningitis. 5. Frontal lobe abscess. 6. Orbital cellulitis and abscess. 7. Cavernous sinus thrombosis.

Chapter 24

duct becomes thickened and polypoidal. Dull headache is an almost constant companion, and, in the worst cases, a state of semi-invalidism is reached.

TREATMENT

Conservative surgery

In the first instance the aim of treatment is to eradicate any infection in the maxillary sinus and ethmoidal cells, and to correct any deformity which impairs the free drainage of the frontal sinus. Thus, antrostomy, or ethmoidal drainage, or submucous resection of the septum, or middle turbinectomy, or a combination of these procedures may be required. In some cases conservative surgery of this nature is successful, but in others it becomes necessary to proceed to more radical operations.

Radical surgery

1   **Radical fronto-ethmoidectory.** A curved incision is made below the medial $\frac{1}{3}$ of the eyebrow and carried down to a point medial to, and below, the inner canthus (Fig. 79). Diseased ethmoidal cells are cleared and a wide channel created to form a new fronto-nasal duct. A tubular skin graft may be inserted in order to preserve patency. An important practical point regarding the preparation for this operation is that the eyebrow should NOT be shaved, for if this is done the patient will present a lop-sided appearance for a very long time.

2   **Obliteration of the sinus** may be resorted to in advanced cases with much bony disease. Techniques vary; some are directed to the removal of the anterior wall of the sinus, others to the raising of an osteo-plastic flap followed by the insertion of the bone chips.

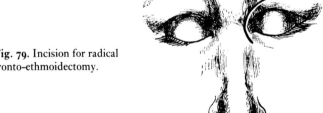

Fig. 79. Incision for radical fronto-ethmoidectomy.

CHAPTER 25
ETHMOIDAL AND SPHENOIDAL SINUSITIS

ACUTE ETHMOIDITIS

ACUTE ethmoiditis is usually present to some extent when the maxillary or frontal sinuses are acutely infected, though in adults it is rare as a separate entity.

In young children it is characterized by redness and swelling below the inner canthus.

Antibiotic therapy is indicated and antral lavage may be necessary.

CHRONIC ETHMOIDITIS

Chronic ethmoiditis is usually associated with chronic infection in other sinuses and is characterized by recurring ethmoidal polypi.

In many cases the maxillary sinus has to be drained and ethmoidal polypi removed from time to time.

In stubborn cases exenteration of the ethmoidal labyrinth, either via the maxillary sinus (Horgan's operation) or externally, may be advised.

SPHENOIDITIS

Sphenoidal sinusitis is rare, and when it does occur is usually associated with infection in other sinuses. The patient complains of severe headache referred to the vertex, retro-orbital or temporal areas; the diagnosis is confirmed by X-rays.

Treatment may include sphenoidal sinus lavage.

CHAPTER 26
SINUSITIS IN CHILDREN

CHRONIC MAXILLARY SINUSITIS

ACUTE infection of the maxillary sinus, with pain and pyrexia, is seldom seen as a clinical entity in children.

Chronic maxillary sinusitis, however, with thick mucopurulent nasal discharge is a common problem.

AETIOLOGY

The infection commences as a complication of nasal foreign body, common cold, tonsillitis, or one of the exanthemata, e.g. measles, and may resolve completely without causing distress. Alternatively, suppuration may linger on for weeks or months if certain predisposing factors are present. These are as follows:

1 Adenoidal hypertrophy.
2 Chronic tonsillar sepsis.
3 Low resistance of the patient, caused by malnutrition, overcrowding, etc.
4 Pulmonary sepsis.
5 The presence of a foreign body.

CLINICAL FEATURES

1 Nasal discharge, often bilateral.
2 Nasal obstruction with mouth breathing.
3 Cough.
4 Tendency to recurrent otitis media and deafness.

EXAMINATION AND INVESTIGATIONS

1 The presence of adenoidal hypertrophy and tonsillar sepsis must be noted.

2 Nasal foreign body must be excluded.
3 Nasal swabs may reveal flora and sensitivity.
4 Transillumination shows opacity of one or both maxillary sinuses.
5 X-ray of sinuses shows opacity or fluid level.
6 X-ray of chest is important to exclude bronchiectasis.

TREATMENT

Nasal vasoconstrictors may be given a trial. The child must be taught to blow his nose (one side at a time), and $\frac{1}{2}$ per cent ephedrine in normal saline drops are instilled 2–3 times daily after nose-blowing. The child should be lying down with the head well back. This method of treatment should not be continued for more than two weeks.

Proetz displacement therapy is applicable to older children, and can be carried out daily by nurse or intelligent parent. The child lies supine with the head far back (chin and external meatal canals in same vertical plane), and is instructed to breathe through his mouth (Fig. 80). 5 cc of $\frac{1}{2}$ per cent ephedrine in normal saline is instilled into the nose, where it remains, submerging the ostia of the sinuses. One nostril is now closed by finger pressure and gentle suction is applied to the other whilst the child says 'K-K-K-K-K . . .', thus sealing the nasopharynx. Air bubbles from the sinuses into the nose, and when suction is interrupted, atmospheric pressure forces solution back into the sinuses. The patient sits up and spits out any nasal discharge and excess solution. By means of this simple treatment inspissated secretions are loosened and ciliary activity stimulated.

Antrum puncture and wash-out is of great value. The child is anaesthetized and placed in the 'tonsil' position.

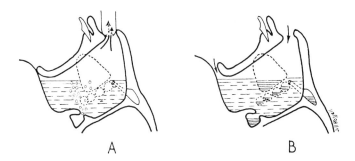

A   B

Fig. 80. Proetz displacement therapy. A. Suction is applied and air leaves the sinuses. B. Atmospheric pressure forces fluid into the sinuses.

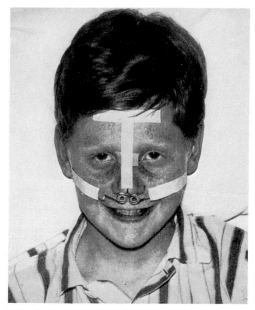

Fig. 81. Walford's silver cannulae have been inserted (under a short general anaesthetic) into the antra, which can now be irrigated painlessly several times daily.

The maxillary sinuses are now punctured and thoroughly flushed with normal saline, washings being referred for bacteriological examination.

Walford's silver cannulae may be left in and the sinuses irrigated painlessly in the ward 3–4 times daily (Fig. 81).

Alternatively, fine polythene catheters may be inserted via metal cannulae. The cannulae are removed, leaving *in situ* the polythene tubes, which are then attached to the face with adhesive strapping.

Intranasal antrostomy is sometimes resorted to in stubborn cases.

Caldwell-Luc operations are avoided if possible in children, in order to avoid risk of damage to developing permanent teeth.

ACUTE ETHMOIDITIS

Acute infection of the ethmoidal cells is occasionally seen in young children and is characterized by redness and swelling below the inner canthus.

Antibiotic therapy is indicated and antral lavage may be necessary.

CHAPTER 27
TUMOURS OF THE NOSE, SINUSES AND NASOPHARYNX

CARCINOMA OF THE MAXILLARY SINUS (ANTRUM)

CLINICAL FEATURES

Early

Carcinoma of the maxillary sinus is seldom diagnosed until the disease has spread to surrounding structures. In its earliest stages it may merely give rise to slight **blood-stained nasal discharge and nasal obstruction.** The patient may have been suffering from chronic catarrh or sinus infection for years, but *the advent of blood in the nasal discharge should give rise to suspicion.*

Late

1 Swelling of the cheek.
2 Swelling or ulceration in the bucco-alveolar sulcus or palate.
3 Epiphora, due to involvement of the naso-lachrymal duct.
4 Proptosis and diplopia, due to involvement of the floor of the orbit.
5 Pain—commonly in the distribution of the 2nd division of the fifth nerve, but may be referred via other branches to the ear, head or mandible.

SPREAD

Local extension is not long delayed. The following may be involved: Cheek, bucco-alveolar sulcus, palate, nasal cavity and naso-lachrymal duct, infra-orbital nerve, contents of orbit, pterygo-palatine fossa (Figs. 82–84).

Lymphatic spread is to the sub-mandibular and deep cervical nodes and is late.

Blood-stream spread is rare.

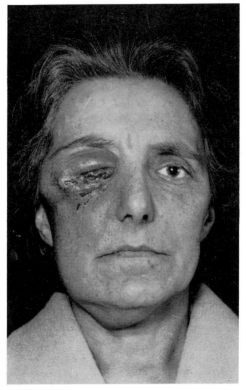

Fig. 82. Carcinoma of the right maxillary antrum. The orbit has been invaded.

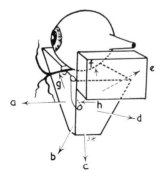

Fig. 83. Local spread of carcinoma of the antrum. *a.* Soft tissues of cheek. *b.* Bucco-alveolar sulcus. *c.* Palate. *d.* Nasal cavity. *e.* Pterygo-palatine fossa. *f.* Orbit. *g.* Infra-orbital nerve. *h.* Naso-lachrymal duct.

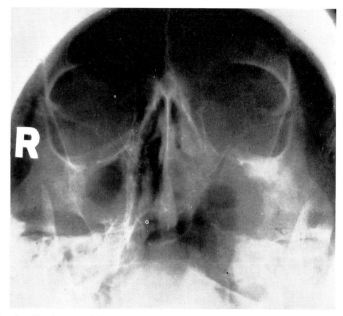

Fig. 84. Carcinoma of the antrum. Note the destruction of the walls of the left antrum. Infection is present in the left frontal sinus and ethmoids.

INVESTIGATIONS

1 X-rays show opacity of the sinus and **destruction** of the bony walls (Fig. 84).
2 Cytological studies of antral washings may reveal malignant cells.
3 Biopsy. A specimen is obtained with punch forceps via the antro-nasal wall, which is often eroded by disease.

TREATMENT

Prior to the development of radiotherapy the most satisfactory method of treatment was by excision of the maxilla.

Now, radiotherapy combined with surgery is the method of choice.

First stage. A full course of tele-radiotherapy is given.

Second stage. The hard palate on the affected side is fenestrated and the patient provided with a dental plate fitted with an obturator (Fig. 85). The cavity of the antrum may now be inspected at intervals and any small recurrence removed by diathermy. In some cases cytotoxic agents may be

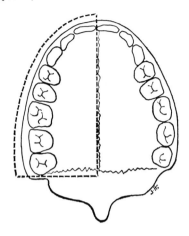

Fig. 85. Fenestration of the palate and alveolus in the treatment of carcinoma of the antrum. The area within the broken line is removed.

used and some years ago the usual method was to infuse the external carotid system with the chosen drug (e.g. methotrexate). The local arterial route is now less commonly employed.

PROGNOSIS

If all figures are considered, only 10–15 per cent of patients can be expected to be alive and well at the end of five years.

CARCINOMA OF THE ETHMOID

The clinical features are similar to those of maxillary carcinoma, but invasion of the orbit and facial skin below the inner canthus is early. Treatment is by radiotherapy.

MALIGNANT DISEASE OF THE NASOPHARYNX

This condition is of interest in view of its geographical distribution and symptomatology. Whereas it is relatively uncommon in Europe (about 1 per cent of malignant cases), it is said to account for no less than 25 per cent of cases of malignant disease in South China.

Pathology. Carcinomata, lympho-epitheliomata, and lymphosarcomata are found.

A small tumour or malignant ulcer in the roof of the nasopharynx infilstrates deeply. Passing through the foramen lacerum, it invades the fifth and sixth carnial nerves, and passing through the pharyngeal wall it invades cranial nerves at the jugular foramen.

Lymphatic spread to the uppermost deep cervical nodes is early and may be bilateral. The enlarged nodes are characteristically wedged between mastoid process and mandible.

CLINICAL FEATURES

Unhappily, some cases of malignant disease of the nasopharynx escape early diagnosis owing to the nature of the presenting symptoms. For example, the patient may complain of deafness and be found to have secretory otitis (as a result of involvement of one or both Eustachian tubes). Or he may present with diplopia (as a result of involvement of the sixth cranial nerve), or enlargement of the cervical lymph nodes.

Such a clinical picture should, but does not always, spell out the possibility of a nasopharyngeal growth and not infrequently cervical lymph nodes have been removed for examination before the presence of the primary growth has been established.

Nasal obstruction and epistaxis may not occur until late and the neurological picture may be complicated by the involvement of combinations of not only the second, third, fourth, fifth and sixth cranial nerves but also the ninth, tenth, eleventh and twelfth.

TREATMENT

Treatment is by radiotherapy. The prognosis in cases receiving early treatment is very uncertain but in late cases is usually poor.

OTHER TUMOURS OF THE NASAL PASSAGES

Osteomata occur in the frontal and ethmoidal sinuses. They are slow growing, and eventually may call for surgical removal.

Nasopharyngeal fibro-angioma. This rare tumour occurs in youths, and causes deafness, nasal obstruction and epistaxis. It is not invasive, but causes serious pressure effects—frog-face, etc. Treatment is by radiotherapy followed by surgical removal, via a palatal incision.

Malignant granuloma, though not truly neoplastic, is a sinister condition characterized by progressive ulceration of the nose and neighbouring structures. There are two main varieties—the *Stewart type*, in which the lesion is limited to the skull and is characterized by a pleomorphic histiocytic infiltration; and the *Wegener type* in which the kidneys, lungs and other tissues may show periarteritis nodosa, the local nasal lesion containing multi-nucleated giant cells. It is probable that malignant granuloma is an auto-immune disease.

Radiotherapy, steroids and cytotoxic agents are used in its treatment, and occasionally are successful.

Malignant melanoma of the nasal septum is of considerable rarity.

CHAPTER 28
NASAL ALLERGY

MECHANISM

SPACE does not permit a full account of the mechanism of the allergic reaction but suffice it to say that in certain individuals reaginic antibodies associated with a class of immunoglobulin designated IgE are present. These, when confronted by allergens (the foreign proteins acting as antigenic substances and ubiquitous in man's environment) promote the liberation of numerous toxic substances including histamine and 5-HT. In turn, increased capillary permeability and vascular dilatation take place with the production of the clinical features of the allergic reaction.

Predisposing factors are as follows:

1 Hereditary. A family history is often present.
2 Psychological. There may be a tendency to psychoneurosis.
3 Hormonal. Sex hormone imbalance may be present.

Allergens may be classified as:

1 Inhalants, e.g. pollens, dusts, powders, moulds and animal emanations.
2 Ingestants, e.g. shell fish, milk, eggs, fruit and certain drugs.
3 Bacteria.

In many cases a pollen of some grass, tree or shrub is the allergen, and such cases are often referred to as **hay fever, pollinosis** or **seasonal** cases. When the allergen is a dust or ingestant the case may be dubbed **non-seasonal** or **perennial**.

CLINICAL FEATURES

Symptoms

1 Rhinorrhoea. The nose pours with clear, watery fluid.

2   Nasal obstruction.

3   Sneezing may be violent and paroxysmal, and is often accompanied by severe irritation of the nose.

4   Conjunctival injection and lachrymation.

Signs

1   Nasal mucosa is thickened and oedematous. It may be abnormally pale or of a bluish tinge.

2   Much clear secretion containing eosinophils is usually present.

3   Sinus X-rays usually show thickened lining of the antral mucosa and sometimes polypi.

INVESTIGATION

The value of careful history-taking cannot be over-emphasized. Any allergen to which the patient may be sensitive should be recorded.

Skin sensitivity tests are often of value. Allergens in high dilution are introduced intradermally by needle or scarifier, and the skin reaction noted.

TREATMENT

Avoidance of contact. It may be possible for the patient to avoid contact with the allergen.

Desensitization. If avoidance of contact is not practicable, a course of desensitizing injections—based on the result of the skin sensitivity tests—is administered. In pollinosis cases, the end of this course should coincide with the commencement of the hay fever season. *In the event of failure the first time, success may attend the same method of treatment in later years.*

Antihistamines are of use in acute attacks. Tolerance is rapidly acquired. The prolonged use of antihistamines should be avoided and patients should always be warned not only that the sedative effect of these preparations may cause a reduction of efficiency in driving and operating machinery but also that this effect is potentiated by C.N.S. depressants such as alcohol.

Vasoconstrictor drops and sprays give relief and may be used sparingly during acute attacks. Their prolonged use is strongly deprecated.

Galvano-cautery applied with care to the mucous membrane of the turbinates produces shrinkage of the thickened tissues, improves the airways and gives some degree of desensitization. It is of particular use in cases where the prolonged use of decongestants has led to almost irreversible changes.

CHAPTER 29
NASAL POLYPI

ETHMOIDAL POLYPI

ETHMOIDAL polypi are common, and cause severe nasal obstruction. They are usually a manifestation of nasal allergy but also result from chronic ethmoiditis (Fig. 86).

Histologically, the polypi consist merely of oedematous musosa, and, macroscopically, they are pedunculated, smooth, pearly or translucent yellow masses. Occasionally they are more fleshy in appearance and may resemble a turbinate. If in doubt, touch with a probe: they are soft, flabby and relatively insensitive, whereas a turbinate is fairly rigid and very sensitive. Treatment consists of removal with nasal snares under topical analgesia or general anaesthesia (Fig. 87). Recurrence is common and in stubborn cases exenteration of the ethmoid may be advised. Short courses of steroids have been advocated for the worst cases.

Children are *rarely* affected by ethmoidal polypi but if nasal polyposis *is* found in a child it may be associated with **cystic fibrosis**. This condition should therefore be kept in mind.

ANTRO-CHOANAL POLYPUS

The mucosal lining of the maxillary sinus (antrum) commonly becomes

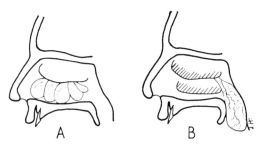

Fig. 86. Nasal polypi. A. Ethmoidal polypi hanging beneath the middle turbinate and obscuring the inferior turbinate. B. A single antro-choanal polypus filling the nasopharynx.

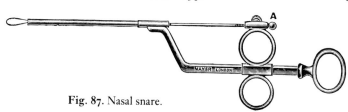

Fig. 87. Nasal snare.

polypoidal as a manifestation of nasal allergy. X-rays clearly reveal polypi lying in the sinus, and *in the great majority of cases so sinus surgery is indicated.*

Rarely, a polypus becomes extruded through the ostium into the nose, and is then known as an **antro-nasal polypus.** Enlarging, it passes back into the choana, becoming an **antro-choanal polypus,** which may then grow to the size of a large walnut and fill the nasopharynx, hanging below the free edge of the soft palate.

Treatment consists of severing the narrow pedicle as it emerges from the sinus ostium; the polypus may then be removed. In recurrent cases the Caldwell-Luc operation is indicated.

CHAPTER 30
NASAL CATARRH

'CATARRH' is one of the most common complaints in the Western hemisphere and embraces such symptoms as nasal obstruction, nasal discharge, post-nasal drip, with repeating clearing of the throat, sneezing and vague headaches.

Though the complaint is of such frequent occurrence, its treatment often leaves much to be desired, for its pathogenesis is but poorly understood by many medical men, the most frequent mistake being to regard all cases of catarrh as due to 'sinusitis' and treat accordingly—with disappointing results.

The most frequent causes of catarrhal nasal symptoms are **vasomotor rhinitis** and **nasal obstructions**. These are therefore dealt with first, and later the less common causes of nasal catarrh are mentioned.

VASOMOTOR RHINITIS

The nasal mucous membrane is the air-conditioning mechanism of the respiratory tract. Its function depends on the delicate balance of its *automatic nervous supply*, and any disturbance of that balance will immediately affect our comfort.

Imbalance may be caused by factors such as **hormonal disturbance** (e.g. during adolescence, pregnancy and the menopause), **anxiety states** or certain **hypotensive drugs**. But unfortunately in the majority of cases no definite aetiological factor can be traced and the patient has to be diagnosed—rather unsatisfactorily—as non-specific **vasomotor rhinitis**.

CLINICAL FEATURES

Symptoms

1 Profuse watery rhinorrhoea.
2 Nasal obstruction.

3   Paroxysmal sneezing.
4   Post-nasal drip.
5   Headache (sometimes).

The symptoms are often of sudden and unexpected onset or they may be maximal on waking, or occur on moving from one atmosphere or climate to another.

Signs

The nasal mucosa is wet and boggy and usually very pale though in some cases it may be of a dusky reddish hue. On X-ray examination the sinuses are found to have a thickened lining mucosa which may be mistaken for evidence of infection. This fallacy in fact—that the most common cause of sinus opacity is infection—is extremely widespread amongst medical men, and has been the cause of countless unnecessary proof-punctures.

It will be seen from the above that the clinical picture closely resembles that of allergic rhinitis and the two conditions are only too often confused. Care must be taken to differentiate between them as the treatment in each case is essentially different.

TREATMENT

Many of the patients who suffer from vasomotor rhinitis are 'vagotonic' individuals who lack exercise and fresh air, tend to over-eat and to 'borrow' heat from central heating, hot baths and thick heavy clothes. **General advice** to lead a somewhat Spartan existence, to lose some weight, and above all to take a sharp walk last thing at night, will often be of value (if implemented). **Ephedrine** by mouth given in increasing dividend doses to a total of 90 mg per diem is often of value. In severe cases **diathermy** of the turbinates or the application of the **cryoprobe** with removal of the hypertrophied posterior ends of the inferior turbinates is of enormous value, and in some cases **vidian neurectomy** is employed. **Vasoconstrictor nasal drops and sprays** are mentioned only to be condemned. Few medicaments in the entire history of therapeutics have been so widely, irresponsibly and unsuccessfully employed as these. Catarrhal subjects seize upon them, attracted by the immediate but transitory relief which they bestow. In many cases a habit forms, and ultimately the nasal mucosa becomes so congested as to fill the nose— 'vasomotor rhinitis medicamentosa'. Rhinologists are not infrequently consulted by patients who have started to use such preparations sparingly but after months or years of regular use almost all vasomotor tone has disappeared from the engorged and turgid nasal mucosa. The unfortunate sufferer, in order to obtain any airway has to resort to his drops or sprays every few minutes and in many cases relief can only be given by diathermy and turbinate trimming under general anaesthesia.

SEPTAL DEFLECTION

Septal deflection, already dealt with in full, is indeed a common cause of catarrhal symptoms. The impaired airway reduces nasal evaporation and excessive mucus finds its way into the nasopharynx (post-nasal drip).

Vasomotor rhinitis may be present in addition to deflected nasal septum and submucous resection of the septum or septal reposition combined with diathermy is the treatment of choice in such cases.

OTHER CAUSES OF NASAL CATARRH

Chronic sinusitis (in adults) is a much less common cause of catarrh than hitherto—owing perhaps, to better living conditions. It must of course be excluded in every case presenting as 'nasal catarrh' and a useful general guide is the macroscopic appearance of the nasal discharge. *A persistently thick green or yellow nasal discharge is likely to be associated with chronic sinus infection.*

Nasal allergy and nasal polypi cause severe catarrhal symptoms; they are dealt with elsewhere.

Catarrh in children is a common problem which (unlike catarrh in the adult) is not infrequently associated with chronic sinus infection secondary to adenoidal hypertrophy. In such cases adenoidectomy and antral lavage is a most salutary form of treatment.

When childhood catarrh is caused by other factors such as allergy or vasomotor instability it is less easy to treat. Psychiatric problems may be involved.

NOTE: *Nasal catarrh may be caused by disordered physiology or by a variety of pathological conditions.*

Forbid your catarrhal patients to use vasoconstrictor drops and sprays.

CHAPTER 31
CHOANAL ATRESIA

CONGENITAL atresia of the posterior nares is caused by persistence of the bucco-nasal membrane, and is, fortunately, rare.

UNILATERAL ATRESIA

One nasal airway is occluded. The condition may pass undiagnosed until the age of 5–10 years, when it becomes apparent that thick mucus is continually accumulating in one side of the nose. On deliberate testing it is obvious that the airway is absent on this side and examination with a probe will reveal a wall of tissue obstructing the airway posteriorly.

Treatment. Exposure of the area is obtained by the transpalatal approach; the obstructing tissue and posterior edge of the vomer are removed with punch forceps, and obturators are used for some weeks or months afterwards.

BILATERAL ATRESIA

This is a much more serious condition. The newly-born infant, deprived of a nasal airway, may be unable to synchronize respiration and degluti-tion, and may die from asphyxia or inanition. There is no time to be lost. Accurate diagnosis must be established by the failure to pass probes or radio-opaque agents from the nose into the nasopharynx.

Treatment in the neo-natal infant is by the nasal route. The membrane is broken down and removed by nasal punch forceps, and the opening is kept patent by tubes. Temporary tracheostomy may be required at some stage.

CHAPTER 32
ADENOIDS

THE adenoid mass of lymphoid tissue is situated on the posterior wall of the nasopharynx and occupies much of that cavity in young children. At the age of about 6 or 7 years, however, atrophy commences, and, as a rule, by the age of about 20 years little or no adenoid tissue remains. In some children of 1–4 years of age, the adenoids, as a result of repeated upper respiratory infections, undergo hypertrophy with the following ill-effects.

Mouth breathing becomes established and results in:

1   Adenoid facies—a narrow nose, prominent incisor teeth, a high arched palate and a perpetually open mouth.
2   Pharyngeal and pulmonary infections.
3   Chronic sinusitis. The normal ventilation and drainage of the sinuses is impaired, with resulting predisposition to infection.

Eustachian obstruction predisposes to:

1   Secretory otitis media with deafness.
2   Recurrent attacks of acute otitis media.
3   Chronic suppurative otitis media.

General manifestations

1   Mental and physical retardation.
2   Snoring.
3   Disturbed sleep.
4   Enuresis.

DIAGNOSIS
The features of adenoid hypertrophy are mentioned above.

The diagnosis is supported by mirror examination of the nasopharynx in the clinic, and by X-rays (lateral view).

In children who are intolerant of examination, the diagnosis may be confirmed by digital or mirror examination under general anaesthesia.

TREATMENT
In most cases of adenoid hypertrophy with persistent mouth breathing, adenoidectomy is indicated. *In cases with aural symptoms, early adenoidec-*

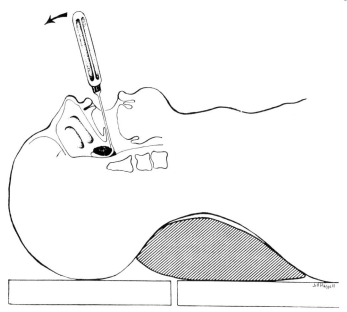

Fig. 88. Adenoidectomy. The curette is swept down the posterior wall of the nasopharynx.

tomy is of supreme importance. Children of 1–3 years of age often benefit by adenoidectomy alone, but in older children much of the clinical picture may be caused by tonsillar sepsis, and tonsillectomy is often performed at the same time.

Adenoidectomy is carried out under general anaesthesia, with the patient in the 'tonsil' position (Fig. 88). An adenoid curette is swept down the posterior wall of the nasopharynx, care being taken to remove all the adenoid tissue and to avoid injury to the Eustachian cushions. A post-nasal pack is left *in situ* for 2 minutes, after which the nasopharynx is inspected with a mirror to ensure that no tags of lymphoid tissue remain. If free bleeding has ceased, the patient is now returned to the ward in a semi-prone position (as in tonsillectomy).

Complications include:
1 Haemorrhage. This usually occurs during the first 24 hours and may necessitate the insertion of a post-nasal plug under general anaesthesia.
2 Otitis media.
3 Recurrence of adenoid tissue.

CHAPTER 33
THE TONSILS AND PHARYNX

ACUTE TONSILLITIS

AETIOLOGY

Acute tonsillitis can occur at any age, but is most common in children under 9.

Spread is by droplet infection, the usual organism being the streptococcus.

CLINICAL FEATURES

Symptoms consist of:

1 Sore throat and dysphagia. Very young children often do not complain of sore throat, but refuse to eat.
2 Earache.
3 Headache and malaise.

Signs

1 Pyrexia may be high and the child is often flushed.
2 Tongue is usually heavily furred. Foetor may be present.
3 Pharynx is hyperaemic.
4 Tonsils are hyperaemic, usually enlarged and exude debris from the follicles—the so-called 'follicular tonsillitis'.
5 Cervical lymph nodes are enlarged and tender.

DIFFERENTIAL DIAGNOSIS

Vincent's angina is characterized by yellowish membrane containing Vincent's organisms, the presence of which can be quickly confirmed by examining a smear.

Scarlet Fever, which is a streptococcal tonsillitis with added features caused by a specific toxin, is very acute in onset, and is characterized by the rash—a punctate erythema—circumoral pallor and a strawberry and cream tongue.

Infectious mononucleosis (glandular fever) may be associated with acute tonsillitis or with membranes featuring Vincent's organisms. Within the first 48 hours the diagnosis may be made with some confidence on account of the mononuclear or lymphocytic leucocytosis; by the end of the first week the Paul Bunnell test is positive.

Diphtheria is more insidious of onset, and is characterized by greyish patches of membrane (which are difficult to remove) on the tonsils, fauces and uvula. Pyrexia is usually low and diagnosis is confirmed by culture— BUT—*if in doubt, treat for diphtheria.*

Agranulocytosis is manifested by ulceration and membrane formation on the tonsils and pharyngeal and buccal mucosa. The neutropenia is characteristic.

TREATMENT

Treatment consists of:
1 Bed.
2 Isolation (within the limits of home-nursing).
3 Copious fluid drinks.
4 Aspirin mixtures.
5 Wool and bandage 'splints' around the neck are very comforting when severe adenitis is present.
6 Antibiotics in severe cases (a satisfactory method is to give one injection of penicillin followed by oral penicillin).

Disinfectant and antibiotic lozenges are of little value and often predispose to monilial infections.

COMPLICATIONS

1 Acute otitis media. (The most common complication.)
2 Peritonsillar abscess (quinsy).
3 Pulmonary infections (pneumonia, etc.).
4 Acute nephritis.
5 Acute rheumatism.

Chapter 33

PERITONSILLAR ABSCESS (QUINSY)

CLINICAL FEATURES

A quinsy is a collection of pus arising outside the capsule of the tonsil in close relationship to its **upper pole**. The abscess occurs as a complication of acute tonsillitis, and is more common in young adults than in children.

The patient, already suffering from acute tonsillitis, becomes **more ill,** has a **peak of temperature**, and develops severe dysphagia with referred otalgia. On examination, a most striking and constant feature is **trismus;** the buccal mucosa is **dirty** and **foetor** is present.

The anatomy of the buccopharyngeal isthmus is distorted by the quinsy, which pushes the adjacent tonsil downwards and medially. The uvula may be so oedematous as to resemble a white grape.

TREATMENT

Systemic penicillin must be given without delay, and in very early cases with 'peritonsillitis' only, abscess formation may be aborted. If much trismus is present and the presence of pus strongly suspected, incision is indicated, for without this, spontaneous rupture may be long-delayed.

Opening a quinsy should be within the province of the general practitioner. The surface of the swelling is lightly painted with 20 per cent cocaine solution, and with the aid of a good light and tongue depressor a

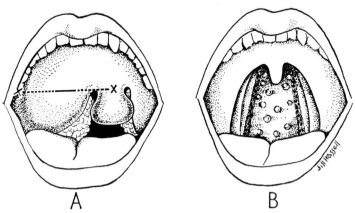

Fig. 89. A. Opening a quinsy. The incision is made midway between the base of the uvula and the site of the upper wisdom tooth on the affected side.
B. Granular pharyngitis, with lateral bands of lymphoid tissue.

small stab incision is made midway between the base of the uvula and the site of the upper wisdom tooth on the affected side (Fig. 89a). A suitable instrument is a pointed scalpel, with all but the terminal $\frac{1}{4}$ inch guarded with adhesive tape.

The blades of a pair of sinus forceps are now inserted into the abscess cavity via this incision, and opened.

The patient spits out pus (and a little blood) and his relief from his previous misery is immediate and dramatic.

In children, general anaesthesia may be necessary, and calls for the utmost skill in its administration.

When a patient has had a quinsy, *tonsillectomy is advised as quinsies are liable to recur*. Many oto-laryngologists prefer to wait 6 weeks before operating, but others operate at the time of the quinsy—'quinsy tonsillectomy'.

RECURRENT TONSILITIS

Some individuals (particularly young children) are subject to recurrent attacks of acute tonsillitis.

Between attacks the patient may be quite symptom-free, and the tonsils appear healthy, or, alternatively, the tonsils may be unduly enlarged and affected by a dull red hyperaemia spreading to the soft palate and fauces. It may be possible to express fluid pus from the crypts. The cervical lymph nodes are often enlarged.

In adults, symptoms such as transient sore throats or a constant tendency to clear the throat are often present, and the condition may be referred to as 'chronic tonsillitis'.

Sinus infections must be excluded. Conservative measures directed to the improvement of the patient's general health may be successful, but, as a rule, tonsillectomy is the only satisfactory method of treatment.

ACUTE PHARYNGITIS

Acute pharyngitis is exceedingly common, and probably commences as a virus infection. It is often associated with acute nasal infections.

The symptoms consist of dysphagia and malaise, and, on examination, the mucosa is found to be hyperaemic.

As a general rule the treatment of acute pharyngitis should consist of regular analgesics such as aspirin 4–6 hourly. Unhappily this complaint is frequently treated by course after course of oral antibiotics often aided and abetted by antibiotic or antiseptic lozenges. As a result the flora of the mouth and pharynx may be completely disturbed and moniliasis ensues with the net result that after 6 weeks of treatment little or no progress has been achieved.

CHRONIC PHARYNGITIS

Chronic pharyngitis may occur as a result of chronic infection of the teeth or sinuses or over-indulgence in spirits or tobacco. Frequently, however, not one of these factors is present.

The most common symptom is discomfort 'in the throat', and a constant tendency to clear the throat.

On examination, there may be the so-called 'lateral bands' of lymphoid tissue, which lie behind the posterior faucial pillars. These bands are more often present in patients whose tonsils have been removed, and are sometimes accompanied by discrete glassy nodules of lymphoid tissue on the posterior pharyngeal wall, when the term 'granular pharyngitis' may be used (Fig. 89b).

An unusual but distinctive form of chronic pharyngitis is keratosis pharyngis, in which white nodular or spike-like aggregations of keratotic material form on the tonsils and pharyngeal wall.

In treating chronic pharyngitis, sepsis and unhealthy habits must be eradicated. Diathermy destruction of lateral bands or lymphoid granules may be necessary, and in keratosis, tonsillectomy is often indicated.

The prolonged use of gargles, sprays and paints is not advised, for the repetition involved in their application serves only to focus the patient's attention on his complaint.

ULCERS AND MEMBRANES OF THE PHARYNGEAL MUCOSA

Ulceration of a mucous membrane is invariably accompanied by a slough which, in some cases, is sufficiently tough to merit the term 'membrane'. The following conditions of ulceration and slough or membrane formation have been alluded to in the differential diagnosis of acute tonsillitis.

1   Vincent's angina.
2   Infectious mononucleosis.
3   Diphtheria.
4   Agranulocytosis.

Other conditions which must also be considered in a case of pharyngeal ulceration or membrane are:

5 Aphthous ulcers. Usually single. White or yellow base. Red surrounding mucosa. History of recurrent ulcers.

6 Moniliasis. White patches of thin membrane. Confirm by smear.

7 Primary syphilis. An indurated ulcer. Gross lymphadenitis. Confirm by smear.

8 Secondary syphilis. 'Mucous patches'. Snail-track ulcers. Confirm by smear.

9 Tertiary syphilis. Ulceration with much destruction. A gumma may perforate the palate or destroy the tonsil.

10 Malignant ulceration. The rolled, everted edge. Induration.

11 Acute tuberculous ulcers. Agonizing dysphagia. Pulmonary tuberculosis is present.

12 Lupus. Painless ulceration and scarring. Rare.

MALIGNANT DISEASE OF TONSIL AND PHARYNX

Carcinoma may occur as an indurated ulcer of the tonsil, fauces or pharyngeal wall. It is often accompanied by earache and slight haemorrhage. Lymphatic spread to the upper deep cervical nodes is early. Diagnosis is confirmed by biopsy.

Lympho-epithelioma and sarcoma tend not to ulcerate, and a sarcoma may provide a diagnostic trap by presenting as a painless hypertrophy of one tonsil.

DICTUM: *In cases of progressive unilateral tonsillar hypertrophy, biopsy or tonsillectomy, with histological examination, is indicated.*

The treatment of malignant growths in this region is by tele-radiation. Prognosis on the whole is poor, though in a small proportion of cases excellent palliation is obtained.

CHAPTER 34
TONSILLECTOMY

THE TONSIL CONTROVERSY

There has always been a curious division of the medical profession into the anti-tonsillectomists and the pro-tonsillectomists. The majority of both camps are well-balanced and moderate in their views but there are 'extremists' who support their cause almost with the fervour of political bigots.

To the extreme 'antis' one should point out that no young child must be allowed to suffer attack after attack of tonsillitis often with otitis media, and the risk of permanent detriment to its hearing or serious toxaemia. Whilst to the 'pros' it must be made clear that tonsillectomy is by no means a trivial operation, and carries with it a small, but undeniable risk. It should not be advised on tenuous indications and without undue consideration.

Judge every case on its own merits.

INDICATIONS

1   Recurrent attacks of acute tonsillitis.
2   One attack of quinsy.
3   Middle ear infection.
4   Cervical lymph node enlargement.
5   Size, causing dysphagia or dyspnoea.
6   Carrier states.
7   Focal sepsis.
8   For histology.

Common indications

The most important and common indication for tonsillectomy is the history of recurrent attacks of acute tonsillitis. Children between the ages of 3 and 8 are particularly susceptible.

One attack of quinsy is likely to be followed by others. The tonsils should therefore be removed after a suitable period (about six weeks) has elapsed.

In recurrent otitis media or C.S.O.M. in children, every attempt must be made to eradicate local sepsis. The adenoids are removed and, in most cases, the tonsils.

Less common indications

If cervical lymph node enlargement persists, infection in the tonsils (perhaps T.B.) must be suspected.

Much fallacy prevails regarding the necessity for tonsillectomy in cases of 'large' tonsils. Nevertheless, they are occasionally so large as to cause dysphagia or even dyspnoea and it is now considered that they have contributed in some cases of 'unexplained' asphyxial death in infancy.

Rarely, tonsillectomy has to be resorted to in carriers of haemolytic streptococci or diphtheria bacilli.

Recurrent attacks of acute rheumatism, nephritis, sinusitis and pulmonary infections sometimes constitute an indication for tonsillectomy.

The patient may be less susceptible to these infections after operation, particularly if the infections are associated with tonsillar symptoms; a good prognosis must not be given with certainty, however, as in a proportion of cases tonsillectomy has little or no effect.

Progressive unilateral tonsillar hypertrophy should be viewed with great suspicion. Malignant disease must be excluded by biopsy or tonsillectomy followed by histological examination.

ADMISSION TO HOSPITAL

During the routine of admission for operation the following questions should be asked:

1 Has the patient had a severe sore throat during the previous month?
2 Has the patient or any relation a tendency to bruise easily or to bleed excessively after minor injuries or dental extractions?

In the event of a recent infection, operation should be postponed, though in some cases of frequently recurring infections, operation under antibiotic cover is decided upon.

If there is the slightest suspicion of any bleeding tendency, the patient should be fully investigated for haemorrhagic disorders. Simple tests for bleeding and clotting time are not adequate.

PREMEDICATION

In children a suitable method is to administer trimeprazine 3 mg. per kilo body weight 2–3 hours before operation, by mouth or 0·9 mg. per kilo intramuscularly. Also, atropine 0·4–0·6 mg. In adults papaveretum 20·0 mg. and atropine 0·6 mg. one hour preoperatively is preferred.

ANAESTHESIA

If rectal thiopentone has been employed, the child is usually asleep on arrival in the anaesthetic room, and nitrous oxide and oxygen, with added ether or Trilene, may be administered without awaking him; psychological trauma is thereby reduced to a minimum.

In adults thiopentone is given intravenously, and an endotracheal tube passed.

Tonsillectomy under local analgesia is feasible, but is practised much less commonly than hitherto.

OPERATIVE TECHNIQUE

The guillotine operation, which, in expert hands, is usually entirely satisfactory, will not be described in detail, as it is preferable for house officers and trainee surgeons to master first the technique of dissection.

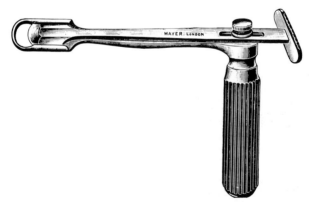

Fig. 90. Heath's tonsil guillotine.

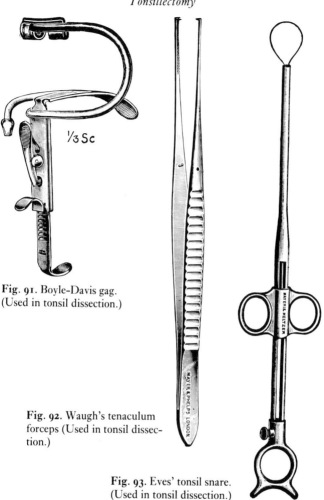

⅓ Sc

Fig. 91. Boyle-Davis gag.
(Used in tonsil dissection.)

Fig. 92. Waugh's tenaculum
forceps (Used in tonsil dissection.)

Fig. 93. Eves' tonsil snare.
(Used in tonsil dissection.)

The **dissection operation** is carried out with the patient lying supine,
the shoulders elevated on a small sandbag. The surgeon, equipped with a
headlamp or mirror, sits at the head of the table.

1   A Boyle-Davis gag (Fig. 91) is inserted, and if adenoidectomy is to be
undertaken the adenoids are removed. In the case of an adult a gauze pack
is inserted around the endo-tracheal tube.

2   The upper pole of one tonsil is firmly grasped with a suitable pair of
tonsil-holding forceps and *drawn towards the mid-line.*

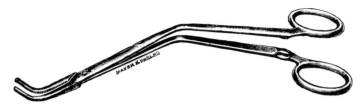

Fig. 94. Wilson's tonsil artery forceps. (Used in tonsil dissection.)

3   An incision is made in the mucosa of the anterior faucial pillar and carried along the anterior and posterior pillars, *keeping as close to the tonsil as possible* (Fig. 95).

4   Further traction of the upper pole towards the mid-line will now open the incision near the upper pole and enable the points of a closed pair of scissors to be inserted.

5   Opening the scissors will now display the capsule of the tonsil, and by using separators, gauze or scissors, the tonsil may be dissected away from its bed. At the lower pole it is usually most adherent, and a snare is used for its final detachment.

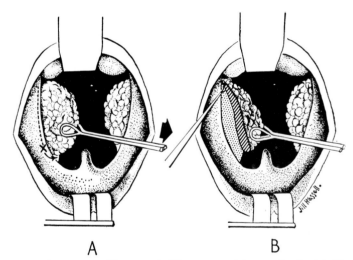

A   B

Fig. 95. Dissection tonsillectomy. A. The mucosa of the anterior faucial pillar is first incised at X. The incision is carried along the anterior pillar (broken line), and also around the upper pole in the direction of the curved arrow, and down the posterior pillar. The broad arrow shows the direction of traction on the upper pole of the tonsil. B. The tonsil has been separated from its bed (stippled), and the lower pole is about to be separated with a snare.

6   The tonsillar bed or fossa is now firmly packed with a wool or gauze swab and the other tonsil removed. Suction is of great value, as haemorrhage may be profuse.

7   All haemorrhage must be arrested before the patient is allowed to leave the table. Vessels are ligated with catgut or thread, using artery forceps (e.g. Wilson's) and Waugh's toothed forceps.

8   Swabs and packs are removed and the swab count verified. The nose and nasopharynx are cleared by suction and the mouth-gag removed. An oral airway is inserted. The patient is turned over into a semi-prone position with a pillow cross-wise under the abdomen and lower ribs.

POST-OPERATIVE CARE

The semi-prone position referred to above is maintained after the patient has been placed in bed, and no pillow is allowed under the head until consciousness has been regained.

The pulse rate is taken every 15 minutes for the first 2–3 hours and then at half-hourly intervals for the rest of the first day.

Responsibility for post-tonsillectomy cases must never be delegated to inexperienced nurses. This is a branch of nursing calling for the highest degree of care, and any untoward event, e.g. haemorrhage, obstruction or rising pulse rate, must be reported immediately, so that necessary action may be taken without delay.

As the reflexes return, the patient starts objecting to—and finally spits out—his metal or rubber airway, then passing into a stage of post-operative sleep.

On awaking, his pillows may be restored to him, and bland fluids, such as orangeade or lemonade, administered. In adults pain may be severe, and pethidine or morphine are justified; nepenthe is of value in children.

The following day swallowing is encouraged, and all but the hardest foods, e.g. crusts or toast, may be given. Great relief from the dysphagia is obtained if a glutinous mixture containing tragacanth and aspirin 600 mg is slowly swallowed by the adult patient about 20 minutes before a meal is due.

Sojourn in hospital—adults 6–7 days, children 2–4 days.

COMPLICATIONS

1   **Haemorrhage** may be reactionary or secondary. Prophylactic measures for its prevention consist of ensuring that (*a*) the patient has no

haemorrhagic tendency, (*b*) the patient has not had a recent throat infection, (*c*) the tonsillar fossae are dry when the patient leaves the operating table.

When haemorrhage does occur, its arrest must be regarded as a matter of urgency. Procrastination may be fatal.

Reactionary haemorrhage occurs within a few hours of operation and is due to rise of blood pressure or slipping of a ligature.

1   Administer a sedative (provided the patient has regained consciousness), take blood for group and cross-match, and with Luc's or similar forceps remove all blood clot from the fossa which is bleeding.

If bleeding is very profuse the patient may have to be taken straight back to the theatre, but in most cases once the clot has been removed the bleeding stops or diminishes.

2   If in 30 minutes bleeding is still present, the patient should be returned to the theatre, re-anaesthetized and the bleeding point ligated.

This dictum may seem drastic, but much valuable time is lost by the repeated application of haemostatic agents, etc., and the patient is in much greater peril if the second anaesthetic has been postponed and his condition weakened by blood-loss.

Secondary haemorrhage occurs between the fifth and tenth postoperative days. It is uncommon but it is the author's practice to warn every adult case, or the parent of every operated child, that it may occur when the sloughs or 'scabs' separate. The warning is coupled with the advice that readmission to hospital is necessary, and indeed very occasionally a minor secondary haemorrhage may be followed by a very serious one within 2 or 3 days.

Usually the only treatment required consists of sedation and careful observation but sometimes a return visit to the operating theatre is necessary. The ligation of a bleeding point in a mass of friable granulation tissue is impracticable, and the haemorrhage is controlled by stitching the faucial pillars together over a small roll of gauze, which is removed 24 hours later (Fig. 96).

FOOTNOTE: With reference to the removal of blood clot in cases of reactionary or secondary haemorrhage it must be stressed that clot should *only* be removed if *active bleeding* is present. The idea of removing clot from a dry tonsillar fossa is of course a nonsense but it is surprising how widespread is this fallacious notion.

2   **Otitis media** sometimes occurs as a complication of tonsillectomy.

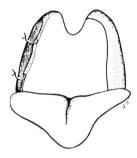

Fig. 96. Severe secondary haemorrhage. The faucial pillars have been sutured together over a small roll of gauze.

Otalgia is present at some stage after almost every tonsillectomy, a fact which is so well known that the unwary may fall into the trap of disregarding the complaint of 'earache' and omit to examine the ears.

DICTUM: *The complaint of earache in a post-tonsillectomy patient calls for an inspection of the tympanic membranes.*

3 **Sepsis.** In some cases marked sepsis is present in the tonsillar fossae and is accompanied by pyrexia, foetor and tenderness in the neck. Secondary haemorrhage is a potential danger, and antibiotics should be given.

4 **Pulmonary complications,** such as pneumonia and lung abscess, are now rare, but lobar collapse occurs from time to time and is evinced by persistent cough, pyrexia and sometimes chest pain. X-ray reveals the site of the collapse, and physiotherapy, combined with antibiotics, effect a rapid cure.

Note: In the preceding chapters the use of aspirin has been advocated on several occasions and it is the author's firm belief that there are few, if any, preparations more appropriate to the relief of the miserable discomfort of a 'sore throat'. Given regularly, aspirin is far more effective than any number of antibiotic, antiseptic or analgesic lozenges, but it is essential that prior to its administration any condition contraindicating its use, e.g. a tendency to peptic ulceration, is excluded.

CHAPTER 35
RETROPHARYNGEAL ABSCESS

ACUTE

AETIOLOGY

The condition occurs, as a rule, in infants or young children. Upper respiratory infection causes adenitis of the **retropharyngeal lymph nodes,** which suppurate. The abscess is limited to one side of the mid-line by the median raphe of bucco-pharyngeal fascia which is firmly attached to the pre-vertebral fascia (Fig. 97a).

CLINICAL FEATURES

The infant or child is obviously ill and has a high temperature. Dysphagia is evinced by dribbling, and there may be stridor. The head is often held to one side. Inspection and palpation of the posterior pharyngeal wall reveal a smooth bulge usually *on one side of the mid-line.*

TREATMENT

Antibiotics should be given in full doses.

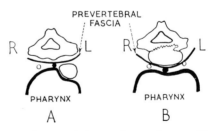

Fig. 97. A. Acute retropharyngeal abscess. A retropharyngeal lymph node on the left side of the median raphe has broken down with abscess formation. B. Chronic retropharyngeal abscess. Cervical caries causing abscess formation behind the prevertebral fascia.

Incision of the abscess, which must not be unduly delayed, is made with the head well down and without anaesthetic.

In an older child a general anaesthetic may be necessary and calls for considerable skill.

CHRONIC

AETIOLOGY

The condition, which affects an older age group, is now uncommon. It is usually the result of tuberculosis of the cervical vertebrae, and the abscess being posterior to the pre-vertebral fascia forms a generalized swelling behind the pharynx (Fig. 97b). *The symmetry of the bulging posterior pharyngeal wall helps to distinguish the chronic from the acute abscess.* Other features of the chronic abscess are the slow development of the condition, and, in most cases, radiological evidence of cervical caries.

TREATMENT

An external incision is made, and the abscess drained after dissection behind the sterno-mastoid muscle and carotid sheath.

CHAPTER 36
THE LARYNX: CLINICAL EXAMINATION:
SOME APPLIED ANATOMY

Indirect laryngoscopy

Before attempting to examine the larynx some skill in the use of the head-mirror for making more simple examinations (e.g. nose and pharynx) should have been acquired. Mirror examination of the larynx calls for patience and gentleness, and the following routine will be found helpful:

1 Choose a laryngeal mirror of 26 mm diameter in the case of a male adult, and 24 mm in the case of a female (Fig. 98). A tarnished mirror should be rejected.
2 Warm the reflecting surface gently and test the back of the mirror on the back of the hand.
3 Instruct the patient to remove his dentures, open his mouth as widely as possible, protrude his tongue and breathe with short panting breaths through the mouth.
4 Wrap the anterior part of the tongue in gauze, protecting the frenulum from the lower teeth, and hold the tongue between the thumb (above) and the middle finger (below). Now, by gently pronating the wrist, the positions of thumb and finger are reversed, and the tongue extruded a little further. *Extreme gentleness is necessary.*
5 Focus the reflected light on the uvula, and holding the mirror like a pencil, pass it into the mouth and press firmly upwards and backwards against the base of the uvula. The mirror must be kept in the mid-line, for any contact with the fauces will induce gagging.

   The patient should be continually encouraged to relax and to maintain his panting respiration; breath-holding predisposes to gagging.

Fig. 98. Laryngeal mirror.

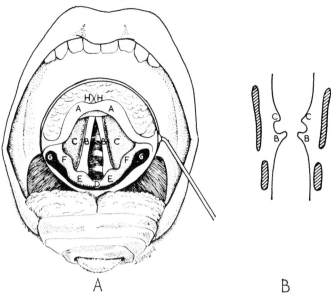

Fig. 99. A. Indirect laryngoscopy. *a*. Epiglottis. *b*. Vocal cord. *c*. Vestibular fold (false cord). *d*. Interarytenoid region. *e*. Corniculate cartilage. *f*. Cuneiform cartilage. *g*. Pyriform fossa. *h*. Vallecula.

B. Diagrammatic coronal section of the larynx, showing the laryngeal sinuses between the vestibular folds above and the vocal cords below.

6   A proportion of patients cannot tolerate the mirror. Do not persist with the examination, but make a further attempt after the patient has sucked a table of Decicain for about 10–15 minutes.

The feature most easily recognized by the novice is the epiglottis, which in some patients is folded to such an extent as to obscure the anterior part of the larynx.

Below the epiglottis (in the mirror image) are the two vocal cords (folds), normally a pearly white hue (Fig. 99). It appears that they are media to, and on the same plane as, the more fleshy vestibular folds, but of course they are in fact on a lower plane.

When considering the familiar mirror image of the larynx it is most helpful to bear in mind a coronal section—a constant reminder of the presence of the laryngeal sinuses between the vestibular folds above and the vocal cords below. Another important fact illustrated by the coronal section is the overhang of the cords, which may obscures a small lesion of the subglottic region.

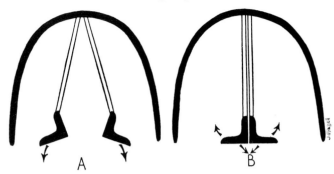

Fig. 100. A. Deep inspiration. The cords are abducted by the posterior crico-arytenoid muscles, which rotate and draw the arytenoid cartilages away from each other. B. Phonation. The cords are adducted by the lateral crico-artenoid and transverse arytenoid muscles.

At the posterior ends of the cords are seen the elevations of the corniculate cartilages, with the interarytenoid region between, and laterally, the cuneiform cartilages buried in the ary-epiglottic folds, which together form the watershed between the air-passage anteriorly and the food-passage behind.

Movements of the cords (Fig. 100)

Ask the patient to breathe in deeply, and note how the cords, which have been in a position of quiet respiration, separate still further and become widely abducted. This is due to the powerful **posterior crico-arytenoid** muscles, which are supplied by the recurrent laryngeal nerves.

Now instruct the patient to sing a long 'E-e-e . . .'. The cords will immediately adduct owing to the action of the **lateral crico-arytenoids** and the **transverse arytenoids**. Their tension is maintained by the

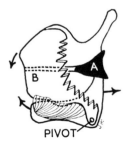

Fig. 101. A. Arytenoid. B. Cord. Contraction of the crico-thyroid muscle increases the distance between thyroid prominence and arytenoid, thereby tensing the cord.

thyro-arytenoid, and by the **crico-thyroid** (Fig. 101), the latter muscle being supplied by the external branch of the superior laryngeal nerve, whilst all the other intrinsic muscles of the larynx are supplied by the recurrent laryngeal nerve.

The hypopharynx

Behind the ary-epiglottic folds (below, in the mirror) is the entrance to the hypopharynx squeezed into a transverse slit by the action of the crico-pharyngeus muscle, which forces the rigid cartilaginous laryngeal box posteriorly, invaginating it into the food passage. At each lateral extremity of the slit is the entrance to the pyriform fossa or lateral food channel. Normally, liquids and semi-solids pass down one or both channels, the hypopharyngeal walls remaining in apposition in the mid-line, but for the passage of a large hard bolus of food the whole lumen of the hypopharynx is necessary, and the laryngeal box is pushed forwards, sometimes with accompanying pain.

In the median line posteriorly, between the strong transverse part (crico-pharyngeus) and the upper oblique part of the inferior constrictor (Fig. 102), is a very weak area—Killian's dehiscence—the site of pharyngeal pouches (diverticula).

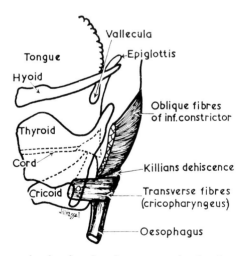

Fig. 102. Diagram showing the crico-pharyngeus embracing the commencement of the oesophagus: the site of Killian's dehiscence is also shown.

The valleculae

Finally, glance back in the upper part of the mirror and inspect the valleculae—two deep recesses separated from one another by the median glosso-epiglottic fold. They lie between the anterior surface of the epiglottis and the tongue and sometimes conceal a small carcinoma.

Fibre-optic laryngoscopy

In some cases a clear view of the larynx cannot be obtained by mirror examination owing to the dentition or the presence of an overhanging epiglottis. Furthermore, some patients defy examination even after the application of local anaesthetic agents. Hitherto it was customary to admit such patients to hospital for direct laryngoscopy under general anaesthesia but the advent of the fibre-optic laryngoscope has made possible the examination of almost every larynx as an out-patient procedure.

CHAPTER 37
INJURY OF THE LARYNX AND TRACHEA

THE larynx and trachea may be injured by:

Penetrating wounds, e.g. gunshot or cut throat injuries.
Blows, e.g. by fists or blunt instruments, or in traffic accidents.
Hot or poisonous vapours—inhaled.
Corrosive poisons—swallowed.
Endotracheal tubes and inflatable cuffs.

Management depends on the severity and extent of the injury. Obviously in a severe case of cut throat, urgent operation will be called for, with the arrest of haemorrhage and, usually, tracheostomy.

In oedema of the glottis, resulting from vapour inhalation or corrosive ingestion, **tracheostomy** may be required.

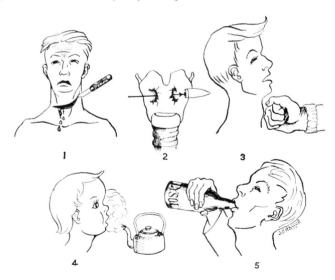

Fig. 103. Laryngeal injury by: 1. Cut-throat or stab wounds. 2. Gunshot wounds. 3. Blows. 4. Inhalation of hot or poisonous vapours. 5. Swallowing of corrosives.

An insidious sequence of events may follow a blow on the larynx, particularly if the cartilages have been fractured. Submucous haemorrhage takes place, causing hoarseness. Glottic oedema gradually increases and **tracheostomy** may be necessary *some hours* after the injury.

In cases of minor injury no active treatment may be required, though vocal rest must be enforced. Where danger of infection of the laryngeal cartilages exists, **antibiotics** are indicated.

Sequelae. Infection→perichondritis→necrosis→fibrosis→laryngeal stenosis.

There is a particular danger of this dismal sequence following penetrating wounds, and, if perichondritis becomes established, fragments of necrotic cartilage may be sequestrated at intervals for months. The laryngeal box becomes shrivelled into a mass of fibrous tissue; the patient is unable to phonate and relies on a tracheostomy for his air-supply.

It is sometimes possible, by external operation and skin-grafting, to restore the laryngeal lumen, thereby avoiding a permanent tracheostomy, but in severe cases little or no voice remains.

NOTE: *Numerous cases of laryngeal and tracheal stenosis have been seen following the prolonged use of indwelling endotracheal tubes. It is well known to the personnel manning intensive-care units that the endotracheal tube in itself constitutes a hazard to the patient and that the type of cuff used and the pressure therein are matters demanding experience and great care.*

CHAPTER 38
ACUTE INFECTIONS OF THE LARYNX

ACUTE LARYNGITIS

Acute laryngitis, more common in the winter months, is usually associated with an upper respiratory infection, such as:

Influenza.
Common cold.
Nasopharyngitis of the exanthemata.

is predisposed to by:

Over-use or mis-use of the voice.
Over-indulgence in strong liquor.
Over-indulgence in tobacco.

If factors from both groups coexist—as, for example, in the foolish individual who, with a severe cold, shouts insults at the gentlemen in the scrum for 80 minutes on a foggy November afternoon—laryngitis is sure to follow.

Clinical features

Aphonia (total loss of voice) or dysphonia (a painful croak).
Pain and tenderness of the larynx. Sometimes.
Other signs of respiratory infection. Sometimes.
Vocal cords pink, oedematous. Traces of mucus.

Treatment

VOCAL REST. This is of supreme importance and is often only achieved by confining to bed.
Bland inhalations of medicated steam (Vap. Benz. or Pini).
Search for and treat any sinusitis or tonsillitis.

ACUTE EPIGLOTTITIS

This condition is a localized infection—usually associated with *H. influenzae* of the mucous membrane of the epiglottis, which becomes congested and oedematous. In the **child** the infection *may kill within hours* by respiratory obstruction and it is now thought that it may have been the cause of some cases of unexplained death in young children in past years.

The practitioner suspecting this infection is advised to seek immediate hospital admission for the young patient for though stridor and respiratory obstruction may be minimal the condition can deteriorate with great rapidity. In **adults** there is severe pain and dysphagia which is usually relieved by antibiotics and analgesics, but death from respiratory obstruction has occurred.

LARYNGO-TRACHEO-BRONCHITIS

This condition occurs in infants and young children. Thick tenacious muco-purulent material forms in the respiratory tract, seriously, and sometimes fatally, curtailing oxygenation.

Treatment

As suggested above, both acute epiglottitis and laryngo-tracheo-bronchitis are dangerous conditions requiring urgent hospital admission. Treatment includes the most careful observation together with oxygenation, massive antibiotic therapy (in some cases chloramphenicol is used) and, in selected cases, steroids. Tracheostomy (q.v.) may be indicated.

LARYNGEAL DIPHTHERIA

Rarely seen now in the British Isles. The child is ill and usually presents the clinical picture of faucial diphtheria. Stridor suggests the spread of membrane to the larynx and trachea.

Treatment

Antitoxin.
General medical treatment for diphtheria.
Tracheostomy (q.v.) may be indicated.

CHAPTER 39
CHRONIC CONDITIONS OF THE LARYNX

Chronic laryngitis.
Laryngeal tuberculosis.
Syphilitic laryngitis.
Keratosis laryngis.

CHRONIC LARYNGITIS

The factors most commonly responsible for the production of chronic laryngitis are as follows:

Habitual shouting as in sergeant-majors, barrow boys, etc.
Faulty voice production found sometimes in teachers, public speakers, ill-trained actors, etc.
Alcohol. (Habitual over-indulgence in spirits.)
Tobacco. (Habitual over-indulgence.)
Chronic sinus infection.

Clinical features

Hoarseness.
Vocal fatigue.
Cough.
Constant tendency to clear the throat.
Nasal obstruction or discharge. (Sinus infection often present.)
On examination:
Cords, and often other soft parts of the larynx, are pink and thickened. Sometimes nodular.

Diagnosis and management

There is a golden rule of laryngology—NEVER MAKE A DIAGNOSIS OF CHRONIC LARYNGITIS UNTIL OTHER LESIONS CAUSING HOARSENESS HAVE BEEN CAREFULLY EXCLUDED.

This may mean X-rays of chest and larynx, serological tests and direct laryngoscopy and biopsy. Nevertheless, chronic laryngitis must not be diagnosed until
Carcinoma of the larynx and hypopharynx,

Laryngeal tuberculosis and syphilis,
Vocal cord paresis,
have been excluded.

When this exclusory process has been accomplished, attention is directed to the eradication of any known aetiological factors, e.g. sinus infection, etc.

Speech therapy is of value when faulty voice production has been a causative factor.

Singer's nodules. These small nodules situated at the junction of the anterior 1/3 and posterior 2/3 of the cords result from vocal strain, and are found, on section, to consist of organized haematomata. They are removed with cup-ended forceps via laryngoscope. Speech training should follow.

LARYNGEAL TUBERCULOSIS

This condition, once common and of serious portent, is now seen much less frequently, thanks to anti-tuberculous drugs. Pulmonary tuberculosis is present, and the first symptom of laryngeal involvement is aphonia or hoarseness due to tuberculous granulations in the interarytenoid region, or ulcers of the cords. Later, agonizing dysphagia may occur. The treatment consists of vigorous attention to the pulmonary disease combined with vocal rest.

SYPHILITIC LARYNGITIS

Syphilitic lesions are much less common than hitherto, but the possibility of a gumma has to be considered in cases of chronic hoarseness in which other lesions have been excluded.

Gummatous infiltration tends to affect the epiglottis and anterior part of the larynx; it may be followed by perichondritis, fibrosis and laryngeal stenosis; it may be accompanied by malignant disease. Anti-syphilitic treatment and, occasionally, tracheostomy are indicated.

KERATOSIS LARYNGIS. (Leucoplakia: hyperkeratosis)

In this condition, almost entirely limited to men, chronic hoarseness is caused by patches of white hyperkeratotic material on the vocal cords.

In some cases the lesion reappears repeatedly after removal, and in time malignant change occurs. The treatment consists of removal of the material with cup-ended forceps via a laryngoscope, and careful histological examination. In recurrent cases removal of the whole cord may be necessary.

CHAPTER 40
TUMOURS OF THE LARYNX

BENIGN

BENIGN tumours of the larynx—papillomata, fibromata and fibro-angiomata—are rare. They occur more commonly in males than in females and cause persistent hoarseness. Small 'granulomata', not strictly neoplastic, sometimes arise as a result of endo-tracheal intubation.

Treatment consists of removal with cup-ended forceps and careful histological examination. The operation is carried out under general anaesthesia using a rigid tubular laryngoscope—this method of examination of the larynx being known as **direct laryngoscopy,** as distinct from indirect laryngoscopy or mirror examination of the larynx, already described. It may be advantageous in many cases to use the operating microscope when performing direct laryngoscopy in which case the procedure is known as *microlaryngoscopy.*

MALIGNANT

Pathology. Almost always squamous-cell carcinoma. *Ten times more common in men than in women (approx.).* Very rarely chondro-sarcoma occurs.

Classification. For many years cases of carcinoma of the larynx were classified as *intrinsic* (on the vocal cords), or *extrinsic* (elsewhere), but this system has fallen by the wayside.

It is now common practice to describe laryngeal tumours in the first place according to their anatomical site as follows:

1 Marginal. (Tip of epiglottis, aryepiglottic folds.)
2 Supraglottic. (Ventricular bands, ventricles, posterior surface of epiglottis, arytenoids.)
3 Glottic. (Vocal cords.)
4 Subglottic. (Below the vocal cords.)

Furthermore, each tumour may be described in terms of the TNM classification to give details of its extent and spread.

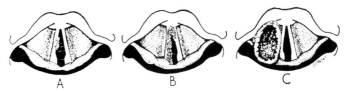

Fig. 104 A. Early glottic carcinoma.
  B. Advanced glottic carcinoma.
  C. Advanced supraglottic growth spreading to aryepiglottic fold.

It is not within the scope of this short book to describe the niceties of the T (Tumour), N (Nodes), M (Metastases) classification but to give examples, a small tumour of one mobile cord with no palpable nodes and no distant metastases would be described as 'Glottic: $T_1 N_o M_o$' whereas an advanced tumour of the supra-glottic region involving a ventricular band, spreading into the epiglottis and associated with homolateral, palpable nodes but with no distant metastases would be dubbed 'Supraglottic: $T_2 N_1 M_o$'.

Symptoms of supraglottic, glottic and subglottic growth. **Hoarseness** is the characteristic symptom and may persist for months before any other symptoms appear. **Dry cough** and slight **haemoptysis** sometimes occur. Later, when the disease has spread and become extrinsic, **dysphagia, dyspnoea** and **earache** may supervene.

Signs. The growth, which may appear as a nodule, an ulcer, a white patch or a fungating mass, is commonly situated, in the case of glottic granules, on the upper surface of the anterior part or middle of the cord. The latter may be fully mobile, sluggish or fixed, any degree of fixation being of serious purport, as it denotes deep infiltration (Fig. 104).

Spread. Local spread takes place:

1 Along the cord to the anterior commissure and into the cord on the other side.
2 Up→vestibular fold→aryepiglottic fold→epiglottis.
3 Down→subglottic region.
4 Deeply→intrinsic muscles.

Lymphatic spread is late, except in the case of supraglottic or subglottic growths, when the deep cervical nodes become involved. Pulmonary metastases sometimes occur. Distant metastases are rare.

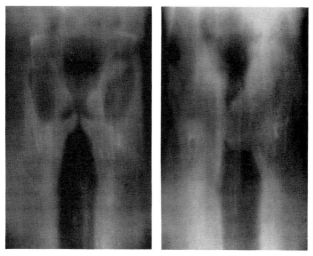

Fig. 105. Tomography of the larynx. The tomogram on the left shows a normal larynx. The tomogram on the right shows a large glottic tumour.

Investigations

1 Direct laryngoscopy or microlaryngoscopy and biopsy.
2 Chest X-ray. (To exclude metastases or T.B.)
3 W.R.
4 Tomography of the larynx (Fig. 105).

Treatment

1 Early cases in which disease is limited to a mobile cord are best treated, in the first place, by **teleradiotherapy** (radium or cobalt unit). In the event of (*a*) failure of the lesion to regress, or (*b*) recurrence, **laryngectomy and block dissection** are indicated.
2 Cases of more extensive disease, with a fixed cord, or cases of subglottic or supraglottic disease, are most safely treated by **total laryngectomy with block dissection** of the cervical lymph nodes.
   The patient will rely on a permanent tracheostomy, but many individuals, with suitable training, acquire the facility of oesophageal speech. Indeed, there are numerous men in varied walks of life, including the professions, who, minus a larynx, carry on their chosen occupation.
3 Late cases, with fixed cervical nodes or local spread to the neck, are

best treated with teleradiotherapy. Good palliation is achieved often, but cure—seldom.

Prognosis

Glottic carcinoma of the larynx, diagnosed early and treated vigorously, has a good prognosis. Diagnosed late, it has a poor prognosis. Never neglect hoarseness.

In marginal cases where the tip of the epiglottis or aryepiglottic folds are affected the symptomatology is less definite, and discomfort or dysphagia are commonly present. Teleradiotherapy may be advised in the first place, but local recurrence frequently takes place, and total laryngectomy, with block dissection, may be advocated. The prognosis is poor.

CHAPTER 41
HOARSENESS: CAUSES AND DIAGNOSIS

CAUSES

Laryngeal

Hoarseness may be caused by any abnormal condition of the larynx—inflammations, neoplasms, pareses, et cetera. The possible causes in each of these categories are numerous, and together they constitute a formidable list.

Pharyngeal

Malignant disease of the oropharynx and laryngopharynx, and pharyngeal pouches, are commonly associated with hoarseness.

General

Hoarseness is sometimes caused by laryngeal oedema and congestion occurring in general conditions, such as myxoedema, renal or cardiac oedema.

DIAGNOSIS

A careful history should always be taken, noting the duration of the hoarseness and the presence of any symptoms suggestive of nasal, pulmonary or other conditions.

Clinical examination includes, in addition to a general examination, an appraisal of the upper respiratory tract with indirect laryngoscopy.

Investigations

Attention has already been drawn to the principle of never making a diagnosis of chronic laryngitis until other lesions have been excluded.

An equally important rule is as follows: HOARSENESS PERSISTING FOR

MORE THAN THREE WEEKS MUST BE INVESTIGATED AND A FIRM DIAGNOSIS
MADE.

The appropriate investigations are as follows:

Chest X-ray.
Tomography of larynx.
Blood Wasserman reaction.
Direct laryngoscopy or microlaryngoscopy and biopsy.

CHAPTER 42
STRIDOR IN INFANTS AND CHILDREN

Congenital cysts, tumours and webs.
Laryngomalacia.
Laryngismus stridulus.
Acute laryngitis.
Acute epiglottitis.
Laryngo-tracheo-bronchitis.
Laryngeal diphtheria.
Multiple papillomata of the larynx.
Foreign body.

STRIDOR in the infant or young child is a clinical sign which must never be ignored. Though some of the conditions causing it are benign, others are rapidly fatal unless relieved by skilled and speedy intervention. The following notes are not intended as full descriptions of the conditions mentioned, and draw attention to their salient features only.

Congenital cysts, tumours and webs may obtrude to such an extent on the airway as to cause immediate asphyxia. When less extensive, stridor is present from birth, and in many cases tracheostomy indicated (Fig. 106a).

Laryngomalacia (Congenital laryngeal stridor). The stridor, which is

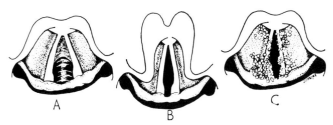

Fig. 106.   A. Congenital web.
             B. Laryngomalacia, a common cause of congenital laryngeal stridor.
             C. Multiple papillomata.

inspiratory, is thought to be caused by abnormally soft and flabby ary-epiglottic folds and epiglottis, the latter in many cases being sharply folded upon itself, forming a perfect valve (Fig. 106b). Stridor is noticed soon after birth and is made worse by feeding or exertion. Tracheostomy is seldom necessary and in most cases of true laryngomalacia the stridor disappears during the first few years of life.

Laryngismus stridulus. Children suffering from rickets or other forms of malnutrition are most often affected. Attacks of laryngeal spasm occur at night, and in severe cases are associated with carpo-pedal contractions and cyanosis.

Traction on the tongue and hot or cold sponging may help to terminate attacks. Between attacks the general health must be attended to.

Acute laryngitis sometimes occurs during whooping-cough or the exanthemata, and may be associated with nocturnal stridor. The use of a steam-kettle and antibiotics usually brings relief.

Acute epiglottitis has already been described as a possible *killer*. Never delay action (see p. 162).

Laryngo-tracheo-bronchitis is also a serious condition calling for expert treatment (see p. 162).

Laryngeal diphtheria. Stridor precedes dyspnoea, and membrane is usually (not always) present on the fauces. The child is ill, with a moderate pyrexia and cervical adenitis. Characteristic foetor is present.

When in doubt give diphtheria antitoxin and penicillin early and in full dosage. Tracheostomy may be necessary.

Multiple papillomata of the larynx sometimes occur in infants and children, and may be of virus origin (Fig. 106c). Repeated removal of the small glassy masses or the application of the cryo-probe is often necessary until puberty, after which recurrence is rare.

Foreign body in the air-passages may cause stridor. A large object impacted in the larynx is likely to necessitate immediate laryngotomy. Smaller foreign bodies in the bronchi are removed endoscopically.

Note: It has already been stressed that stridor in an infant or child calls for extreme care and circumspection in its management. It is a sign which denotes respiratory obstruction and we must never lose sight of this fact or, indeed, the possibility that it may herald a vicious circle terminating in death.

It is sometimes said that many young children 'grow out' of a tendency to stridor but this is a dangerous attitude. *Every case of stridor should be investigated.*

CHAPTER 43

VOCAL CORD PARESIS

Nerve supply of the laryngeal muscles

All the intrinsic muscles of the larynx, with the exception of the crico-thyroids, are supplied by the recurrent laryngeal nerves.

The *crico-thyroids*, which act as tensors of the cords, are supplied by the external branches of the *superior laryngeal nerves*.

Semon's law. *In a progressive lesion of the recurrent laryngeal nerve, the abductors are paralysed before the adductors.* Thus, in incomplete or partial paresis, the cord will be brought to the mid-line by the still active adductors, but when paralysis is complete, it moves away a little to the so-called paramedian position. Semon's law has never been fully understood. For many years it was considered that the abductors were more vulnerable than the adductors owing to their later evolution. Opinion is now divided on this point though the fact remains that as a rule the abductors do seem to be affected first in progressive lesions.

Left recurrent nerve paresis (Fig. 107) is a relatively common

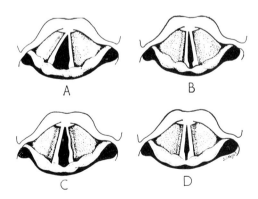

Fig. 107. A. Left recurrent nerve paralysis (inspiration).
B. Left recurrent nerve paralysis (phonation).
C. Left combined paralysis.
D. Bilateral abductor paralysis on deep inspiration.

condition and is associated in the early stages with a weak, high-pitched voice. Later, as the contralateral cord compensates, the voice improves. The causes are as follows:

In the chest:

> Carcinoma of the bronchus.
> Carcinoma of the oesophagus.
> Malignant mediastinal nodes and primary neoplasms.
> Pulmonary tuberculosis and its surgery.
> Aortic aneurysm.
> Cardiac hypertrophy and cardiac surgery.
> Penetrating wounds.
> Peripheral neuritis.

In the neck:

> Carcinoma of the thyroid gland.
> Trauma during thyroidectomy.
> Malignant cervical lymph nodes.
> Carcinoma of the hypopharynx and oesophagus.
> Penetrating wounds.

Right recurrent nerve paresis is much less common. The causes are the same as for the left nerve, but are confined to those sited in the neck. Tuberculous thickening of the apical pleura, once a fairly common cause of paresis of the right nerve, is seen less frequently.

Bilateral recurrent nerve paresis (bilateral abductor paralysis) most commonly occurs as a result of thyroidectomy or malignant disease of the thyroid gland or neck. A similar condition is sometimes seen in rheumatoid arthritis, when there may be crico-arytenoid joint ankylosis. In any of these conditions the airway may be seriously endangered. Why? Refer back to Semon's law. When there is a partial paresis of **both** nerves, and **both** cords lie in the mid-line, asphyxia is imminent, and tracheostomy may be necessary. Later, when the paralysis becomes complete, the airway may be adequate except during exertion.

Combined superior and recurrent nerve paresis occurs in lesions of the medulla or the vagus above the origin of the superior laryngeal nerve. Clinically, the cord is flabby owing to loss of tone in the crico-thyroid. Commonly, the paresis is bilateral, when the associated sensory loss (internal laryngeal branches) increases the chance of inhalation pneumonia. The causes are as follows:

Medulla—Bulbar poliomyelitis, syringobulbia, vascular and neoplastic lesions.

Vagus trunk—Tumours of the base of the brain and in the region of the jugular foramen, e.g. carcinoma of nasopharynx.

Functional aphonia is almost limited to females. The patient speaks in a whisper for periods of days or months at a time. On mirror examination it is clearly seen that the cords will not adduct if the patient is asked to say 'E . . . e . . . e', but if she is asked to cough the cords adduct perfectly!

The treatment of vocal cord paresis

The cause should be found if possible and the appropriate treatment given. Speech therapy is of great value in strengthening the voice in unilateral cases. In bilateral cases permanent tracheostomy may be required, and patients fitted with a K.C.H. valve tube often phonate extremely well. Numerous operations have been devised to abduct one cord, thereby rendering permanent tracheostomy unnecessary.

Functional aphonia is best treated by reassuring the patient (having carefully excluded organic disease) and referring her to a speech therapist. Psychiatric advice is sometimes necessary.

CHAPTER 44
CONDITIONS OF THE HYPOPHARYNX

Foreign bodies
Chronic hypopharyngitis
Malignant disease
Pharyngeal pouch
Non-organic 'throat discomfort'

FOREIGN BODIES (Fig. 108)

Fish, poultry and other bones are often inadvertently swallowed, and, in most cases, scratch or tear the hypopharyngeal mucosa, but pass down into the stomach and are eventually voided. Sometimes, however, they become impacted in the hypopharynx or oesophagus, and unless removed may lead to perforation, parapharyngeal abscess or mediastinitis, and even fatal perforation of the aorta.

Management

The casualty officer in a hospital of average size may be called upon several times a week to decide whether or not a patient complaining of a bone in the throat is in fact harbouring a foreign body or has discomfort resulting from a scratch due to the recent passage of a foreign body. Patients with such abrasions of the mucosa in the post-cricoid region steadfastly assert that the bone is still present.

The following routine should be adopted:
1   Take a careful history, noting the nature of the suspected foreign body (? radio-opaque) and the time of ingestion.
2   Examine the pharynx and larynx, paying particular attention to the fauces and tonsils (herring or kipper bones often stick here).
3   X-ray the neck and chest.
4   If marked dysphagia is present or a foreign body is seen on X-ray, oesophagoscopy is indicated.
5   If symptoms are slight and X-rays are normal, see the patient daily until symptom-free, but if symptoms persist oesophagoscopy is indicated. The potential gravity of an oesophageal foreign body cannot be over-

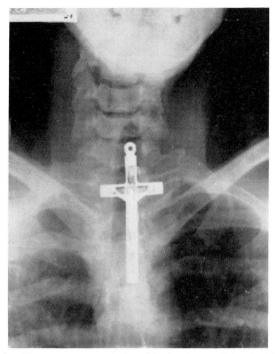

Fig. 108. An object most commonly found in the chest wall, but in this unusual case firmly wedged in the cervical oesophagus. A *very* large oesophagoscope was required.

emphasized, and in the continued presence of symptoms normal X-rays must NOT be allowed to give rise to a feeling of security. Laryngologists are only too familiar with tragic fatal cases, or records of such cases, which at some stage have been lightly passed off as 'only a swallowed fish bone'.

CHRONIC HYPOPHARYNGITIS

The Paterson-Brown Kelly or Plummer-Vinson syndrome occurs in middle-aged women.

Symptoms

1   Gradually increasing dysphagia.
2   Loss of weight.
3   Soreness of tongue and lips.
4   Fatigue.

Signs

1 Angular stomatitis.
2 Chronic superficial glossitis.
3 Koilonychia (spoon-shaped nails).
4 Microcytic anaemia.
5 Atrophy of the hypopharyngeal mucosa with cracking, bleeding and the formation of webs.

Some cases are steadily progressive, and eventually a **post-cricoid carcinoma** arises in the atrophic mucosa of the hypopharynx.

Treatment

The anaemia must be treated vigorously. Dysphagia due to hypopharyngeal webs may be relieved by periodic dilatation.

MALIGNANT DISEASE (Fig. 109)

Malignant disease of the hypopharynx occurs in two main forms:
1 Carcinoma of the pyriform fossa, or lateral food channel—predominantly a disease of **men.**
2 Carcinoma of the post-cricoid region—predominantly a disease of **women.**

Clinical features

The chief symptoms are **increasing dysphagia** and **loss of weight.** Some women patients admit to dysphagia or 'small swallow' over a period of years, suggesting that the Paterson-Brown Kelly syndrome has been present.

A lump in the neck may be the first complaint of a man with a lesion

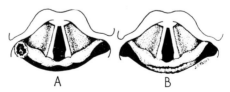

A   B

Fig. 109. Malignant disease of the hypopharynx.
A. Pyriform fossa.
B. Post-cricoid.

the size of a sago grain in the pyriform fossa, not yet causing dysphagia but active enough to have spread to the regional nodes, where there is a swelling the size of a pigeon's egg. **Hoarseness** may be due to involvement of the recurrent laryngeal nerve, and referred **otalgia** is sometimes present.

On mirror examination, the upper edge of a malignant ulcer may be clearly seen, but more often the only sign of a lesion is a pool of saliva in the pyriform fossa. In many cases no abnormality is apparent.

Spread

Spread locally into the neck and to the deep cervical lymph nodes is early. Pulmonary and distant (e.g. suprarenal) metastases sometimes occur.

Investigations

Barium swallow is invariably indicated in cases of dysphagia, and if any abnormality is detected oesophagoscopy must be undertaken without delay.

It is important to note that a negative barium swallow does not necessarily exclude disease, and if symptoms persist oesophagoscopy must still be performed.

Treatment

Laryngopharyngectomy with block dissection of cervical lymph nodes and replacement by stomach or colon is the only treatment which gives any chance of a lasting cure. It is, however, limited to fit patients without distant or fixed local metastases, and even in such cases the recurrence rate is high.

Radiotherapy, though capable of good palliation in cases of pyriform fossa carcinoma, is extremely disappointing when applied to post-cricoid growths.

In advanced cases of malignant disease of the hypopharynx **tracheostomy** and **gastrostomy** are sometimes indicated, and no effort must be spared to relieve the patient's misery with **analgesics, sedatives** and **tranquillizers.**

PHARYNGEAL POUCH (Hypopharyngeal diverticulum (Fig. 110))

These are herniations of mucosa through Killian's dehiscence—the weak area between the oblique and transverse fibres of the inferior constrictor. It is thought that the predisposing cause is muscular incoordination. Pharyngeal pouches occur most commonly in elderly males.

Clinical features

1   Discomfort in the throat, when pouch is small.
2   Dysphagia, as pouch becomes larger.
3   Regurgitation of undigested food.
4   Gurgling noises in the throat. Sometimes.

Investigation is by barium swallow and oesophagoscopy.

Treatment. In the early case with a very small pouch operative treatment may be averted by periodic dilatation of the oesophagus; the object being to stretch the powerful muscle fibres of the cricopharyngeus, which impede the onward progress of the food bolus, but more advanced cases (as for example in Fig. 110), require surgery. Via a neck incision, and

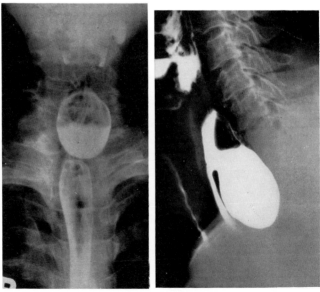

Fig. 110. Two views of a hypopharyngeal diverticulum containing barium.

with careful dissection, the pouch is removed and the hypopharyngeal defect carefully sutured after which a myotomy of cricopharyngeus (transverse fibres of the inferior constrictor) is performed. Dohlman's method or endoscopic diathermy of the thin party wall between the oesophagus and the diverticulum is of particular value in old and feeble patients who are unsuitable subjects for major surgery.

NON-ORGANIC 'THROAT DISCOMFORT'

Every year medical practitioners, and particularly laryngologists, are approached by numerous patients who complain of fairly persistent discomfort in the throat.

Various terms are used by the patient in an attempt to describe the symptoms—'A piece of cotton-wool or apple-peel' or 'a hair lodged in the throat' or, simply 'a lump in the throat'. But on questioning, these patients scarcely ever admit that there is any interference with swallowing, in fact they often volunteer that they are only free from symptoms at meal times.

The number of such patients attending rises steeply whenever the media draw attention to throat cancer in a prominent person and sometimes patients shamefacedly confess that their symptoms commenced after the death of a relative or close friend from malignant throat disease. There is invariably an element of anxiety.

For very many years the condition of non-organic throat discomfort has been referred to as *'globus hystericus'*, but in the author's view it is a dangerously facile term and has all too often been wrongly applied to patients in the early stages of organic disease. The management in such cases is to take a careful history, examine the patient and order a barium swallow.

Patients are usually reassured by negative findings but, remember, a 'negative' barium swallow does not invariable rule out organic disease and if symptoms persist endoscopy under general anaesthesia will be necessary.

CHAPTER 45
TRACHEOSTOMY

TRACHEOSTOMY, or the making of an opening into the trachea, has been practised since the first century B.C., and is an operation which any medical man may be called upon to perform.

INDICATIONS

There are many indications, which may be classified as follows: (1) conditions causing upper respiratory obstruction, (2) conditions necessitating protection of the tracheo-bronchial tree, and (3) conditions causing respiratory insufficiency.

UPPER RESPIRATORY OBSTRUCTION

Congenital.	Choanal atresia.
	Laryngeal webs and cysts.
	Stenosis of the trachea.
	Tracheo-oesophageal anomalies.
Trauma.	Gun-shot and cut-throat laryngeal injuries.
	Blows on larynx.
	Inhalation of steam or poisonous gases.
	Swallowing of corrosives.
Infections.	Acute epiglottitis.
	Laryngo-tracheo-bronchitis.
	Diphtheria.
	Ludwig's angina.
Tumours.	Advanced malignant disease of tongue, larynx, pharynx or trachea.
	Radiotherapy in carcinoma of larynx (sometimes causes oedema).
	An adjunct to surgery in carcinoma of larynx.

Carcinoma of thyroid gland, hypopharynx or
cervical lymph nodes.

Laryngeal paralysis. Following thyroidectomy.

Bulbar palsy.

Rheumatoid arthritis.

As a temporary measure to cover operations
for the relief of bilateral vocal cord paralysis.

Foreign body.

PROTECTION OF THE TRACHEO-BRONCHIAL TREE

Many conditions are a source of danger to the respiratory epithelium by
facilitating the inhalation of saliva, food, blood or gastric contents. Tracheostomy enables the tracheo-bronchial tree to be aspirated at frequent
intervals, and also permits the continued use of a cuffed-tube, which may
be necessary in some cases.

Bulbar poliomyelitis.

Myasthenia gravis.

Polyneuritis.

Tetanus.

Coma due to: head injuries.

barbiturate poisoning.

cerebral vascular catastrophes.

cerebral tumours.

cerebral surgery.

diabetes.

uraemia.

eclampsia.

cardiac arrest.

Multiple fractures of the jaws.

Burns of the face.

RESPIRATORY INSUFFICIENCY

Tracheostomy in cases of respiratory insufficiency is of value for the
following reasons:

1   Reduction of dead space (lips to tracheostome).

2 By-pass of glottic resistance.
3 Aspiration of secretions from the tracheo-bronchial tree.
4 Administration of warmed and humidified gases.
5 Maintenance of controlled respiration (in some cases).

The conditions leading to respiratory insufficiency may be considered under the following headings:
1 Pulmonary disease.
2 Abnormalities of the thoracic cage.
3 Neuro-muscular dysfunction.

Pulmonary disease

Exacerbation of chronic bronchitis, with emphysema.
Post-operative pneumonia with suppression of cough.

Abnormalities of the thoracic cage

Severe chest injury ('flail chest').

Neuro-muscular dysfunction

Many conditions have already been cited as indications for tracheostomy for the purpose of protecting the tracheo-bronchial tree from inhaled secretions. Tracheostomy is also necessary in some of these conditions, e.g. deep coma, for the application of intermittent positive pressure respiration (I.P.P.R.).

Wet-lung syndrome. In some cases several factors are present and augment each other to build up a rapidly fatal condition—the 'wet-lung' syndrome (Fig. 111).

CRITERIA FOR PERFORMING TRACHEOSTOMY

How does one know that the moment has arrived when conservative measures must be abandoned and tracheostomy performed?

In the obstructive cases there may be stridor, and recession at the suprasternal notch and supraclavicular, intercostal and epigastric regions. The patient will be anxious, restless, sweating and pale. Cyanosis denotes that a late stage has been reached, and the accessory muscles of respiration may be functioning.

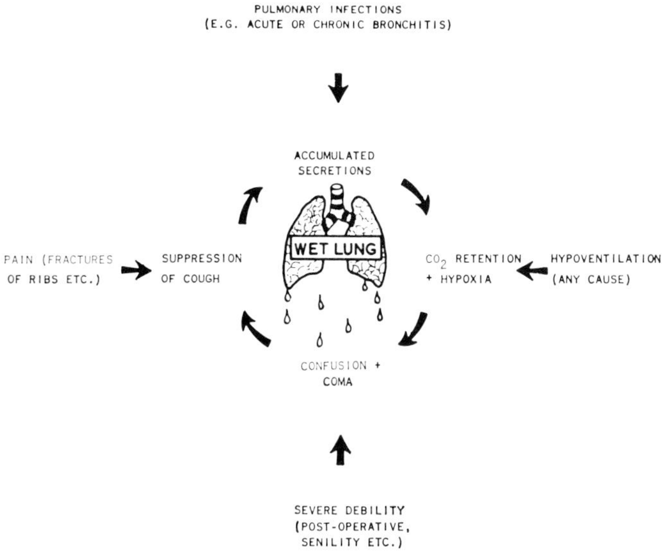

Fig. 111. In some cases of respiratory insufficiency several factors augment each other, producing a rapidly fatal condition—the 'wet-lung' syndrome.

Do not wait for this grim picture to develop, for by waiting, incalculable damage will be done.

In the non-obstructive cases tracheostomy should be carried out as an *elective procedure*, not resorted to in desperation.

DICTUM: *In cases of respiratory obstruction or respiratory in sufficiency, and in the absence of steady improvement—perform tracheostomy.*

TECHNIQUE

Anaesthesia. In past years tracheostomy was almost always performed under local analgesia. Today it is more often performed under general anaesthesia after preliminary intubation. A high degree of skill is required.

Position. The patient lies supine with the head hyperextended over a small sandbag placed under the neck.

Infiltration. The subcutaneous tissues of the neck are infiltrated in the incisional area with 0·5 per cent Lignocaine.

Incision. A 5 cm. transverse collar incision, the mid-point of which is midway between the cricoid cartilage and suprasternal notch, is carried down to the investing layer of deep cervical fascia (Fig. 112).

Investing layer and pretracheal muscles are now separated by a vertical mid-line incision and held apart by broad Langenbeck retractors.

Pretracheal fascia between the cricoid cartilage and thyroid isthmus is now incised, exposing the first ring of the trachea. The trachea should be carefully palpated to confirm its position.

Thyroid isthmus is lifted (by blunt dissection) away from the trachea and divided between clamps, exposing the second, third and fourth tracheal rings.

The tracheal window is now made by resecting a circular area of the anterior wall of the trachea, including portions of the second and third or third and fourth cartilaginous rings. A vertical or cruciate incision alone is inadequate. *A disc of tissue must be removed.*

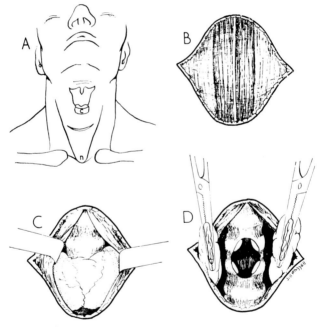

Fig. 112. Tracheostomy.

    A. The incision is midway between the cricoid cartilage (*c*) and suprasternal notch (*n*).

    B. The investing layer of fascia covering the pretracheal muscles.

    C. The thyroid isthmus.

    D. The tracheal window.

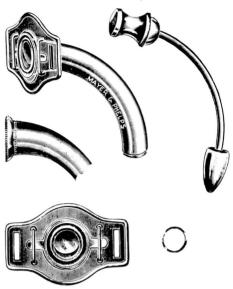

Fig. 113. Negus' (K.C.H.) tracheostomy tube.

Choice of tube. A good example of silver tube is the K.C.H. pattern (Fig. 113), which combines many admirable features. The Durham tube, which has an adjustable flange, is of value in emaciated patients where the skin-trachea distance is small, or in very obese patients where the corresponding distance is great (Fig. 114).

When intermittent positive pressure respiration, or protection of the lungs from pharyngeal secretions, are necessary, a cuffed tube must be employed.

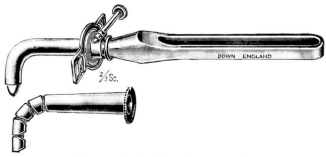

Fig. 114. Durham's tracheostomy tube.

Insertion of tube and closure of wound. The trachea is now aspirated and the tube inserted. Bleeding points are ligated. The wound is *loosely closed* by one of two sutures on either side of the tube. Closing the wound tightly and in layers courts disaster by facilitating surgical emphysema or by impeding the reinsertion of an accidentally displaced tube.

AFTER CARE

Nursing care must be of the highest order. The patient should not be left for at least 24 hours.

Position. The patient should be well propped-up in bed.

Suction is applied at regular intervals, and the rubber catheter should pass down into the trachea and main bronchi.

Humidification of inhaled air may be achieved by the use of a steam-kettle, humidifier, or moistened gauze placed over the external end of the tube.

Softening of secretions is essential and is aided by Alevaire in the form of a spray or Lomudase insufflations.

Tube changing. The inner component of a silver tube may have to be removed for cleansing at hourly intervals during the first 24 hours. The whole tube should not be removed for 5–6 days. Cuffed rubber tubes require special attention, e.g. regular deflation of the cuff.

Extubation (when tracheostomy seems no longer necessary) should be carried out only when the patient is able to sleep serenely with the tube corked.

COMPLICATIONS

Perichondritis and laryngeal stenosis may follow if the cricoid cartilage is injured. *Go below the first ring.*

Mediastinal emphysema may occur after a very low tracheostomy. *Do not go too low. Do not close the wound tightly.*

Obstruction of the tube or trachea by crusts of inspissated secretion may prove rapidly fatal. *If suction fails to produce a clear airway act boldly.* Remove the tube and search for the obstruction with forceps; an explosive expiration will now eject the crust as from a gun, and the tube may be replaced.

Complete dislodgement of the tube may occur if the tapes are not secured reasonably firmly around the patient's neck. The wound edges and track should be held apart with tracheal dilators until a clean tube is replaced.

Partial dislodgement of the tube is a sinister complication which may terminate fatally. The inner end of the tube is dislodged from the tracheal lumen and takes up a position adjacent to the innominate artery. After a period of hours or days a catastrophic haemorrhage takes place. PROPHYLACTIC MEASURE—*ensure that at all times the patient is breathing freely through the tube.*

LARYNGOTOMY

Students having read a detailed description giving the various stages of tracheostomy often ask (or should ask): 'How can I, when a relatively inexperienced doctor, be expected to perform this difficult operation under appalling conditions in a welter of blood, on an asphyxiating patient with only a pen-knife?'

The question is a valid one and conjures up the dramatic scene of a man staggering out of a pub and falling to the ground, his airway completely obstructed by a pickled onion impacted in the laryngeal inlet. Two minutes from death. What to do?

Forget tracheostomy. Run the finger-tip down from the Adams apple to the depression between the thyroid and cricoid cartilages and having found this depression plunge in the knife with the blade poised horizontally taking care to keep in the midline. Here the airway is nearer the skin than at any other point and in the words of Negus this life-saving operation of laryngotomy or crico-thyrotomy may be done *in a few seconds.*

As soon as the knife has entered the airway, the thyroid and cricoid cartilages are prized apart and some sort of improvised tube inserted. It must be emphasized that no patient should be left with a laryngotomy for more than an hour or two, as there is a risk of perichondritis of the laryngeal cartilages with the sinister end-result of laryngeal stenosis. The airway having been restored by emergency laryngotomy, tracheostomy is now performed *under good conditions,* and the laryngotomy incision closed.

CHAPTER 46
DELUSIONS AND FALLACIES

THAT 'quick-acting' ceruminolytic ear-drops never cause trouble (see p. 27).

That ear drops are satisfactory as the sole treatment in otitis externa (see p. 31).

That headache is likely to accompany uncomplicated otitis media (see p. 54).

That secretory otitis—a common condition—could not have a grave underlying cause (see pp. 59 and 125).

That earache must be caused by some form of ear disease (see Fig. 53).

That pills will cure tinnitus (see p. 69).

That patients will respond happily to being told to 'learn to live with' their tinnitus (see p. 69).

That almost every form of giddiness may be referred to as 'Menière's Syndrome' (see p. 70).

That mothers can always be cheerfully reassured that their young children have normal hearing (see p. 78).

That sudden deafness can be 'sat upon' (see p. 78).

That a fractured nose may wait almost any length of time before it has to be reduced (see p. 92).

That nose bleeding cannot be serious (see p. 99).

That the operation of S.M.R. is still the only method of correcting a deflected nasal septum (see p. 101).

That swellings of the face are commonly due to sinus infection (see p. 109).

That a course of desensitizing injections which has apparently failed in the treatment of hay fever is 'not worthwhile' repeating (see p. 128).

That antihistamine drugs may be distributed *ad lib* (see p. 128).

That a common underlying cause of 'nasal catarrh' is sinusitis (see p. 132).

That the majority of nasal symptoms such as rhinorrhoea are the result of sinusitis (see p. 132).

That X-ray opacities of the maxillary antrum invariable denote infection (see p. 133).

That vasoconstrictor drops and sprays should be employed in the treatment of nasal catarrh (see p. 133).

That mild attacks of 'sore throat' are best treated by antibiotics (see p. 141).

That tonsillectomy is either 'in-fashion' or 'out-of-fashion' (see p. 144).

That tonsillectomy is a relatively trivial operation and post-operative cases may be delegated to inexperienced nurses (see p. 149).

That clots should be removed from tonsillar fossae under all circumstances (see p. 150).

That indwelling endo-tracheal tubes are free from hazard (see p. 160).

That a stridulous child may be nursed at home—with confidence (see p. 162).

That persistent hoarseness is an insignificant symptom (see p. 169).

That a child who has stridulous attacks will probably 'grow out' of them and need not be investigated (see p. 172).

That a swallowed fish bone is a triviality (see p. 177).

That a negative barium swallow can be relied upon to exclude disease in the hypopharynx and oesophagus (see p. 179).

That tracheostomy is a simple operation (see p. 189).

CHAPTER 47
EXAMINATION QUESTIONS

As stated in the preface to the first edition, the study of past questions is a 'must' if a candidate expects to do well in any examination. When confronted with the paper remember the following tips:

1 Apportion your time carefully, leaving adequate time at the end to read through your answers.

2 Read the questions very carefully. Candidates in the heat of battle sometimes fail completely to perceive part of a question.

3 Answer the questions without padding and concentrate on facts. But make sure you get the facts right. Headings and subheadings are welcomed by hard-pressed examiners, who are not amused by page after page of homogeneous prose.

4 If asked to give a number of symptoms, signs, complications, methods of treatment, etc., always deal with the important and common items first. If you are sure you have all these in—then go on to the small-print stuff, but not before.

5. One or two simple diagrams, if appropriate to the subject, may be of help in clarification, BUT do not waste time on elaborate works of art. It is unlikely that these will be appreciated by posterity.

SURGERY

The following questions have been set in the surgery papers of the final examinations for medical and surgical degrees of the Universities of Cambridge (C), London (L), and Oxford (O), and the final examinations for LRCPLond, MRCSEng (Conj.).

1958. For what conditions would you perform tracheotomy? Give your reasons and describe the operation (C).

Write brief notes on (a) acute glaucoma, (b) acute frontal sinusitis, (c) acute suppurative otitis media (C).

Discuss the indications for tonsillectomy (L).

Write short notes concerning: (*a*—*d*) *d*, Pharyngeal pouch (Conj.)

1959. Describe briefly how you would deal with the following conditions occurring in a country practice: (*a*—*e*), *b*, Earache (C).

1960. Discuss the oesophageal lesions causing slowly increasing dysphagia (L).

Give an account of the diagnosis and treatment of acute otitis media (O).

Write short notes on: (*a*—*d*), *c*, Otitis media (Conj.).

Write short notes on the following: (*a*—*c*) *c*, Maxillary sinusitis (Conj.)

Write short notes on the following: (*a*—*d*) *b*, Otitis externa (Conj.).

1961. Give an account of the symptoms and signs associated with disease of the maxillary antrum (L).

Describe the complications of infection of the middle ear, and their treatment (L).

Describe the symptoms and signs of maxillary sinusitis (O).

Write short notes on the following: (*a*—*d*) *d*. Quinsy (Peritonsillar abscess). (Conj.).

Discuss the differential diagnosis and treatment of acute otitis media in a child. (Conj.).

1962. Write short notes on: (*a*—*e*) *a*. Quinsy (C).

Write an essay on the surgical relief of deafness. (Choice of four other subjects. Duration: $1\frac{1}{2}$ hours.) (O).

1963. What are the causes of epistaxis? (O).

Write short notes on: (*a—d*) *a*. Frontal sinusitis. (C).

Give the indications for tracheostomy. Describe the post-operative care of the patient. (C).

Write short notes on the following: (*a—d*) *d*. Frontal sinusitis. (Conj.).

Write short notes on the following: (*a—d*). *d*. Retropharyngeal abscess. (Conj.).

Discuss the differential diagnosis of dysphagia. (Conj.).

Describe the facial nerve. What types of paralysis occur? (Conj.).

Write short notes on the following: (*a—d*). *c*. Otitis media. (Conj.).

1964. Give an account of the diagnosis and complications of chronic suppurative otitis media. (L).

Discuss the causes and investigation of dysphagia in a woman of 50. (L).

Tabulate the causes and treatment of epistaxis. (O).

Write short notes on: (*a—e*) *a*. Infection in the maxillary antrum. *b*. Facial nerve palsy. (C).

Write short notes on: (*a—d*) *a*. Earache in a child of 6. (C).

Write short notes on: (*a—d*) *c*. Epistaxis. (Conj.).

Describe the trachea and its relations. Give the indications for tracheostomy. (Conj.).

1965. How would you investigate a patient presenting with a unilateral nasal discharge? (L).

Give the causes and appropriate treatment of epistaxis. (O).

Write short notes on: (*a—e*) *a*. Quinsy. (C).

Write short notes on: (*a—e*) *c*. Otitis Externa. (C).

Write short notes on: (*a—d*) *c*. Oedema of the glottis. (Conj.).

1966. How would you investigate a patient with a discharging ear? (L).

What are the common causes and treatment of deafness? (O).

Write short notes on: (*a—e*) *c*. The maxillary antrum. (C).

Write short notes on: (*a—e*) *a*. Earache in childhood. (C).

Write short notes on: (*a—d*) *c*. Epistaxis. (Conj.).

Write short notes on: (*a—d*) *a*. Otitis externa. (Conj.).

Describe the anatomy of the trachea and discuss the complications of tracheostomy. (Conj.).

MEDICINE

The following questions have been set in the **medicine** papers of final examinations.

1958. A woman of 45 complains of difficulty in swallowing. Discuss the investigation and management. (Conj.).

1959. Discuss the diagnosis of severe pain in one side of the face. (Conj.).

1960. Discuss the indications for tracheostomy. (Conj.).

Name five causes of difficulty in swallowing, and mention two additional findings of diagnostic importance. (Conj.).

1961. How would you assess the significance of vertigo in a middle-aged woman? (L).

Give (*a*) Five conditions causing absence of knee-jerks with extensor plantar responses. (*b*) Five causes of facial palsy. (Conj.).

All the following are side effects of drugs; in each instance name the drug and one condition for which it is used.

(*a—j*) *d*. loss of balance. *f*. tinnitus. *g*. deafness. (Conj.).

List five causes of stridor in childhood and indicate one appropriate treatment in each case. (Conj.).

1962. Discuss the medical indications for tracheostomy. (L).

1963. What is the connecting link between (*a—j*)? *h*. facial nerve palsy and aural discharge. (O).

Discuss the causes of dysphagia in a woman of 55. (C).

For each of the following name one drug likely to be the cause. (*a—j*) *a*. Tinnitus. *b*. Vestibular damage. (Conj.).

Define as for a concise dictionary: (*a—e*) *c*. Menière's syndrome. (Conj.).

A man aged 45 becomes hoarse: discuss the possible causes. (Conj.).

How is stridor produced? Discuss the differential diagnosis. (Conj.).

1964. Discuss the possible cause of vertigo. How would you investigate such a case? (L).

What is the link between anaemia and: Dysphagia, Hoarseness (eight other clinical features mentioned). (Conj.).

Name two drugs which may cause (*a—e*). *b*. Deafness. (Conj.).

1965. Discuss the differential diagnosis of a sore throat. (L).

Give an account of the causes of vertigo. How would you investigate this condition in a man of 60? (L).

A woman aged 35 complains of dysphagia. What might be the matter with her? (L).

Describe in detail the treatment of acute tonsillitis in a boy of 7 years. List the complications. (Conj.).

1966. What is Bell's palsy? Describe its clinical features and treatment. (L).

A mother complains that her child of 3 years is not yet talking. Discuss the differential diagnosis. (L).

What are the causes of dysphagia in a woman of 55? (C).

Note: In the questions on dysphagia, all causes, cervico-thoraco-abdominal, must be taken into consideration. In the question 1960 (L), post-cricoid and pyriform fossa lesions should be included in the answer, though they are not strictly oesophageal.

CHAPTER 48
FURTHER READING AND HIGHER
QUALIFICATIONS

The author is very conscious of the fact that in the foregoing chapters the subject of otolaryngology is treated in barest outline. It is hoped that owners of enquiring minds have not been excessively frustrated by this necessarily brief account, but if so they are advised to consult the following excellent works.

BALLANTYNE J.C. (1977) *Deafness*, 3rd ed. London, Churchill.

SCOTT-BROWN W.G., BALLANTYNE J.C. and GROVES J. (1979) *Diseases of the Ear, Nose and Throat*, 4th ed. London, Butterworth.

MAWSON S.R. and LUDMAN H. (1979) *Diseases of the Ear*, 4th ed. London, Arnold.

WILSON T.G. (1962) *Diseases of the Ear, Nose and Throat in Children*, 2nd ed. London, Heinemann.

BULL T.R., RANSOME J. and HOLDEN H. (1979) *Recent Advances in Otolaryngology*, 5th ed. Edinburgh, London and New York, Churchill Livingstone.

BALLANTYNE J.C. and GROVES J. (1978) *Synopsis of Otolaryngology*, 3rd ed. Bristol, John Wright.

MORRISON A.W. (1975) *Management of Sensorineural Deafness*. London, Butterworth.

In studying for higher qualifications, reference to the following journals will also be necessary.

The Journal of Laryngology and Otology
The Journal of the Royal Society of Medicine
Acta Oto-laryngoligica
The Annals of Otology, Rhinology and Laryngology
Archives of Otolaryngology
Laryngoscope.

HIGH QUALIFICATIONS
Diploma in Laryngology and Otology (D.L.O.)
This diploma is offered by the Royal College of Physicians of London and

the Royal College of Surgeons of England. The examination is in two parts, both of which are held every six months.

Part I consists of the basic sciences of otolaryngology and Part II is concerned with clinical work. The D.L.O. is a useful stepping-stone in the specialty but should not be regarded as the ultimate academic achievement by the novitiate in otolaryngology.

Fellowship of the Royal College of Surgeons (F.R.C.S.)

The Royal Colleges of Surgeons of England, Edinburgh and Ireland and the Royal Colleges of Physicians and Surgeons of Glasgow offer diplomas of Fellow in Otolaryngology. Regulations vary from time to time and from one College to another and prospective candidates are advised to seek up-to-date regulations from the appropriate College.

The regulations relating to the examinations for the diploma of Fellowship of the Royal College of Surgeons of England (and for the D.L.O.) may be obtained from The Secretary, Examination Hall, Queen Square, London WC1.

Degree of Master of Surgery (M.S., M.Ch., Ch.M.)

Many of the universities offer Masterships in Surgery which may be conferred following the presentation of a satisfactory thesis, either in general surgery or in a branch of surgery such as otolaryngology. In some cases the candidate is required to sit an examination as an alternative to or in addition to submitting a thesis but here again regulations vary and details must be sought from the academic registrar of the university concerned.

INDEX

Mastoid cells, 2
Mastoidectomy, cortical, 43, 49, 50
  epitympanic, 43
  radical, 43
Mastoiditis, acute, 46
  zygomatic, 47
Meatus, external auditory. *See* External auditory meatus
Melanoma of the nasal septum, 126
Membranes of pharynx, 142
Menière's disease, 70
Meningitis in frontal sinusitis, 115
  in middle ear infection, 49
Microcytic anaemia, 178
Microlaryngoscopy, 165
Mirror, head, 85
  laryngeal, 154
  post-nasal, 87
Molars, impacted, as a cause of earache, 67
Moniliasis, 141, 143
Mononucleosis, infectious, 139
Mouth breathing in children, 136
Multiple papillomatosis of the larynx, 172
Myringoplasty, 44
Myringotomy in acute otitis media, 38
  in secretory otitis media, 58, 59

Nasal allergy, 127
Nasal bones, fracture of, 91
Nasal catarrh, 132
Nasal diphtheria, 104
Nasal discharge in acute maxillary sinusitis, 109
  carcinoma of antrum, 121
  choanal atresia, 135
  chronic maxillary sinusitis, 110, 118
  nasal allergy, 127
  nasal diphtheria, 104
  vasomotor catarrh, 132
Nasal furunculosis, 104
Nasal obstruction in adenoids, 136
  carcinoma of antrum, 121
  carcinoma of the nasopharynx, 125
  choanal atresia, 135
  nasal allergy, 127

nasal polypi, 130–131
septal deflection, 100
septal haematoma, 93
septal perforation, 103
sinusitis, 109, 110
vasomotor catarrh, 132
Nasal osteomata, 125
Nasal packing, 96
Nasal polypi, 130–131
Nasal septum. *See* Septum, nasal
Nasal vasoconstrictors, 109, 119, 128, 133
Nasal vestibulitis, 104
Nasopharynx, clinical examination of, 85
  malignant disease of, 124
Nephritis in tonsillitis, 139
Nodules, Singer's, 164
Nose, clinical examination of, 85
  deformity of, 91, 93, 102
  foreign body in the, 89
  injuries of, 91
Nose-picking, 103
Nystagmus, in caloric tests, 71
  in cerebellar abscess, 54

Oedema of the glottis, 159
Oesophageal speech, 167
Orbital complication of frontal sinusitis, 115
Osteomata of the sinuses, 125
Osteomyelitis of frontal bone, 115
Otalgia (Earache), 65, Fig. 53, 67, 151
Otitis externa, 28
Otitis media, acute, 35–39
  chronic, 40–45
  complications of, 46
  facial palsy in, 83
  following tonsillectomy, 150
  secretory, 57
Otomycosis, 28
Otorrhoea in acute otitis media, 37
  in carcinoma of the meatus, 33
  in chronic otitis media, 40
  in mastoiditis, 47
  in otitis externa, 29
Otosclerosis, 61